HISTORICAL DANCES
FOR THE THEATRE

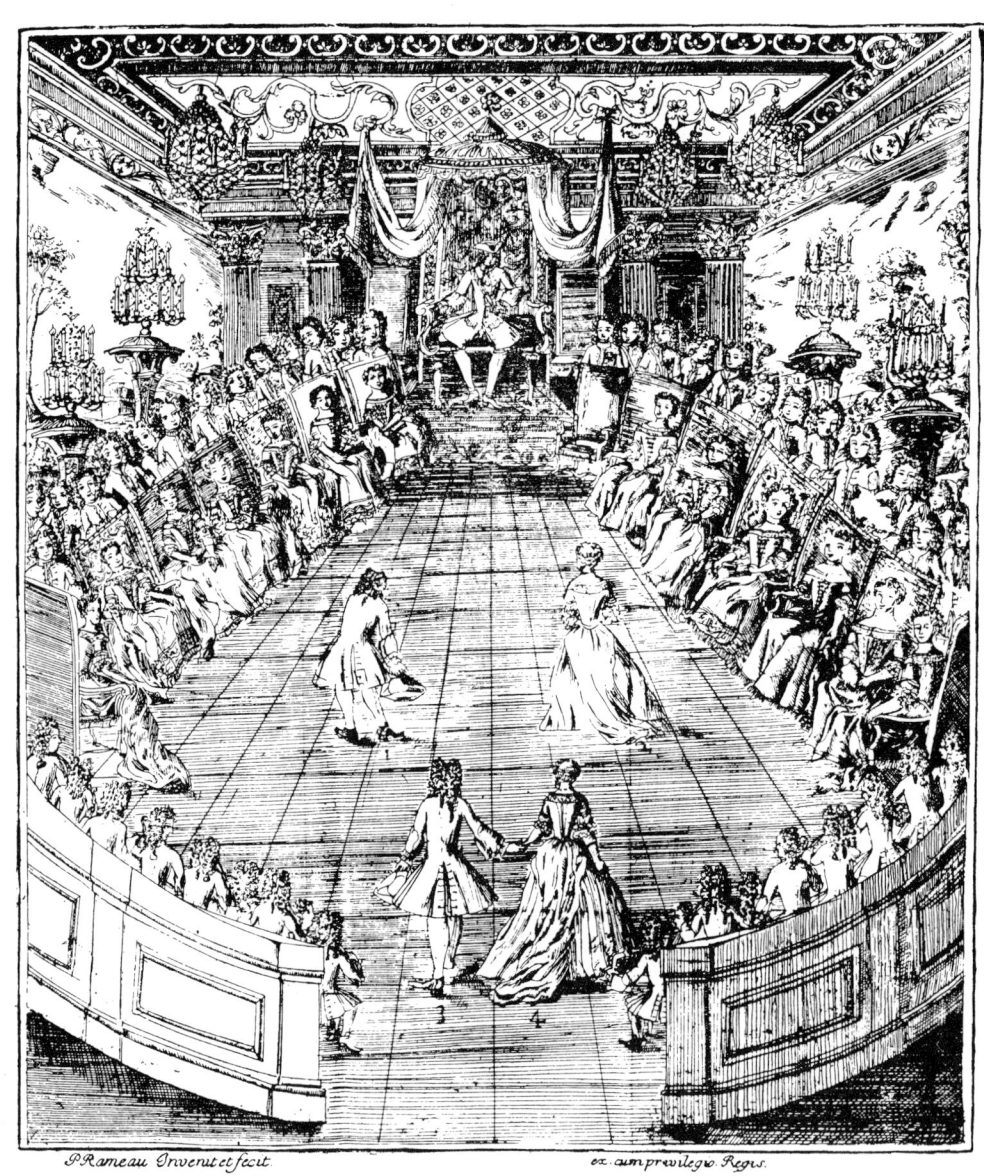

(From 'Le Maître a Dànser' by P. Rameau)

HISTORICAL DANCES FOR THE THEATRE

The Pavan and the Minuet

by

JOHN GUTHRIE

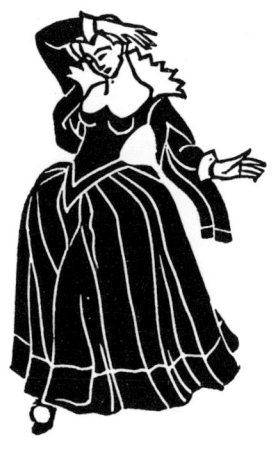

Dance Books Ltd
9 Cecil Court, London WC2

To Mrs. Arnold Dolmetsch

©1982 John Guthrie
First published 1950,
this edition published 1982 by
Dance Books Ltd.,
9 Cecil Court, London WC2N 4EZ

ISBN 0 903102 68 4

AUTHORS' NOTE

THIS BOOK, the result of many years of practical work and careful research, was written and completed in the Autumn of 1938 and the Spring of 1939, the intention being that it should be the first of a series of textbooks on the dances of the fifteenth, sixteenth and seventeenth centuries; the whole forming a complete and authoritative work for professional dancers and choreographers. The outbreak of war, however, and years of military service made it quite impossible for me to continue the project. Whatever is added to these studies must be left to another generation of students.

Venice, May, 1949.

ACKNOWLEDGMENTS

To Mrs. Arnold Dolmetsch, the original inspiration, teacher and good friend for twenty-three years.
To Mrs. Oswald Powell (Margaret), for many years of close collaboration and patient research.
To Mrs. George Carley, for her kindness in preparing the music.
To my father, James Guthrie, for planning and supervising the printing of the book.

CONTENTS

	PAGE
Introduction	1
Behaviour and Deportment in the Ballroom	5
The Bow or Reverence	7

THE PAVAN

History	8
Music	11
Steps	11
Figures	13

THE MINUET

Part One: History

General Nature of the Minuet	14
Origins	16
The Golden Period	21
Further Developments	23

Part Two

How to Dance the Minuet	26
Music	26
Tempo	27
The Minuet Step	27
French Style, Forwards	28
Backwards	28
Sideways to the Left	28
Sideways to the Right	29
English Style,	29
Forwards	29
Backwards and Sideways	29
The Passepied Step, or the Fleuret and a Bound	30
Ornamental Steps	30
The Contretemps	30
The Balancé	32
The Flying Bourrée	32
The Double Bourrée	33
The Coupée or Marchés	33
The Slip and Half Coupée	34

CONTENTS (*continued*)

	PAGE
Minuet Step and Ornamental Steps: Later Period	34
The Pas Grave, Forwards	34
Sideways	35
The Fleuret	35
The Balancé, Forwards	35
Sideways to the Right	37
Turning to the Right	37
Pas de Mons. Marcel	37
Arm Movements for the Minuet Step	39
Presenting of Arms	42
Ornamental Steps	42
Observations on Style	44
The Double Honours	48
Summary of the Feuillet Dance Notation in Relation to the Minuet	49
Foot in Air Sign	49
Turning Signs	49
Bends, Bounds and Hops	49
Rests	50
The Fifth Position	50
Notation	
Table of Signs used in describing the Minuet	53
Minuet Step, French Style	54
English Style	54
Ornamental Steps, Early Period	55
Later Period	57
Diagrams of the Minuet	56, 58 to 63
Music	
Pavana Bray, William Byrd	67
Pavan, Luys Milan, 1635	69
Minuet, Eighteenth Century, English	72
Deux Passepieds, Jean Joseph Mouret, 1730	74
Bibliography	79

INTRODUCTION

BEFORE *proceeding with the real purpose of this book, the author feels that some sort of apology is necessary for adding yet another work to the already extensive collection of books on the dances of the past, to say nothing of the books for 'balletomanes' that have appeared within the last few years.*

In Victorian times it was fashionable to produce histories of dancing, and it was found possible to include a survey of the whole history of the art, ranging from the ritual dances of the early Egyptians down to the polka, the pictures being chosen, with astonishing impartiality, from the works of Botticelli or Maud Goodman, according to which dance seemed to need illustration. A certain superficiality of treatment, inseparable from this manner of approach, deprives these histories of any real value for the purposes of the professional dancer of to-day.

Again, in our own time, there seems to be a tendency for the antiquarian aspect to be stressed unduly; and, while the question of whether a certain dance originated in the ritual of human sacrifice, or as a means of bringing rain, in some dim past, is no doubt of interest to the sociologist, it is of very little use to the dancer, who only wishes to know how the dance was performed; an aspect of the subject about which the antiquarian can tell him nothing.

The subject of old dances as a possible source of inspiration to the modern choreographer has never been more than superficially explored, although certain eminent choreographers of our time have made use of the more obvious and accessible material. As a general rule, the professional dancer has very little time to undertake laborious research work, nor is he always fitted for it by temperament or training; and, as choreographers are usually primarily dancers, the same holds good for these also. They work, unconsciously, with a repertoire of movements and a technical foundation, which is centuries old, and without which their art would not exist. Yet the cry of the young choreographers is always 'Let us do away with everything that belongs to the past, and start afresh'. The result is that modern ballets, set in a past time, usually show the most extraordinary misconceptions of how people danced and moved in those days.

It is not the purpose of this book to go into critical details of the modern ballet; but it is worth noting that Michel Fokine's ballet, 'Don Juan', is a striking example of an almost complete misunderstanding of the execution of sixteenth and seventeenth century dances—whether purposely or unwittingly, I am unable to say.

A slavish reproduction of these early dances is not necessarily the ideal to be striven for, but a proper understanding and appreciation of them ARE necessary before departing from the original form. Here the question may be asked whether we have not advanced too

HISTORICAL DANCES FOR THE THEATRE

far to make it worth while recalling these dances with the comparative simplicity and lack of variety which must surely characterise them. Anyone, however, who has performed or witnessed any of the dances of the periods under consideration, will readily agree that they are fully worthy of reconstruction, both for their own beauty, and as sources of inspiration.

The sixteenth century Italian schools alone provide a rich store of romantic and beautiful dances, with the most varied and captivating music imaginable. Fabritio Caroso, the Venetian dancing master, gives no fewer than seventy-eight varieties of gagliarde, cascarde, balletti, etc., in his book, 'Il Ballarino' (1581); and Thoinot Arbeau, the Canon of Langres, gives directions for a great number and variety of dances in his book, 'Orchesographie' (1588); enough for many years' study and practice. This does not take into account other contemporary authors, or the fifteenth century bassedanses, or the innumerable seventeenth century collections of chaconnes, passacailles, entrées, gigues, etc.

That the music was almost always of great beauty is not to be wondered at, when it is understood that nearly all the great composers wrote dance music along with other musical forms. As a result, we have in the sixteenth century, besides the adaptations of popular songs and airs, pavans and galliards by William Lawes, bassedanses by Pierre Attaignant, and balletti by Horatio Vecchi, to name only a few. The seventeenth and eighteenth century composers are too well-known to need mention here, but it is worth remarking that the standard declined rapidly from the middle of the eighteenth century. The words and dance music of the succeeding period are mostly insipid and banal. The Industrial Revolution was probably responsible for this decadence, as for many another. In our own time, popular dance music, despite its many supporters, has few enduring qualities; and it is hard to imagine our more exclusive composers setting themselves to the business of producing foxtrots and rumbas for the West End ballrooms and cabarets, except from what might be termed motives of 'inverted highbrowism'.

The difficulties surrounding the elucidation and true interpretation of the early dance forms are innumerable, and a great deal of general study and experiment is necessary before even the simplest of them becomes clear. A wide knowledge and appreciation of the manners and social customs of the periods under consideration help materially in arriving at the style in which the dances were originally performed. It is worse than useless to have the steps correctly executed with the arm movements derived from modern ballet, or without arm movements at all, as is the practice of some of our modern schools of dancing.

The old dancing masters were not always very explicit in their directions, and ambiguities present themselves at every turn, often at vital points; or so it seems. To make things more obscure, they had no exact technical terms, such as the Five Positions of the feet and arms

INTRODUCTION

used in classical ballet to-day. Occasionally they were not very clear themselves how certain steps were to be done. Arbeau goes so far as to write, with reference to the steps of the Canaries, that 'You will learn them from those who know them, and you can invent new ones for yourself'—a delightfully naive confession of ignorance that does little towards describing the dance. The eighteenth century masters only seem to be more lucid because the dances they were describing are nearer to our own kind, and their technical terms are more akin to our own. Cyril Beaumont has a word of caution for the student on this point, in the introduction to his excellent translation to P. Rameau's 'Maître à Danser' (1752). He writes, 'When the dance student meets with a familiar technical term, there is a not unnatural tendency to interpret it in the light of modern technique, with which the student is doubtless familiar. Nothing could be more fallacious or more apt to produce difficulties where none exist. The student should do no more than carry out the author's instructions, for, although many eighteenth century steps bear familiar names, as regards their manner of execution, they frequently differ considerably from their modern equivalents.' The same, in a lesser degree, may be said of the dances of earlier centuries.

The foregoing will give the reader some idea of the difficulties that have to be overcome before a little book of this kind becomes at all possible; but he is, happily, not directly concerned with them, and has only to make use of the results as far as he is in need of them. The author hopes, with all humility towards his predecessors in the past centuries, that he has succeeded in making his descriptions clear and concise enough for all practical purposes.

HISTORICAL DANCES FOR THE THEATRE

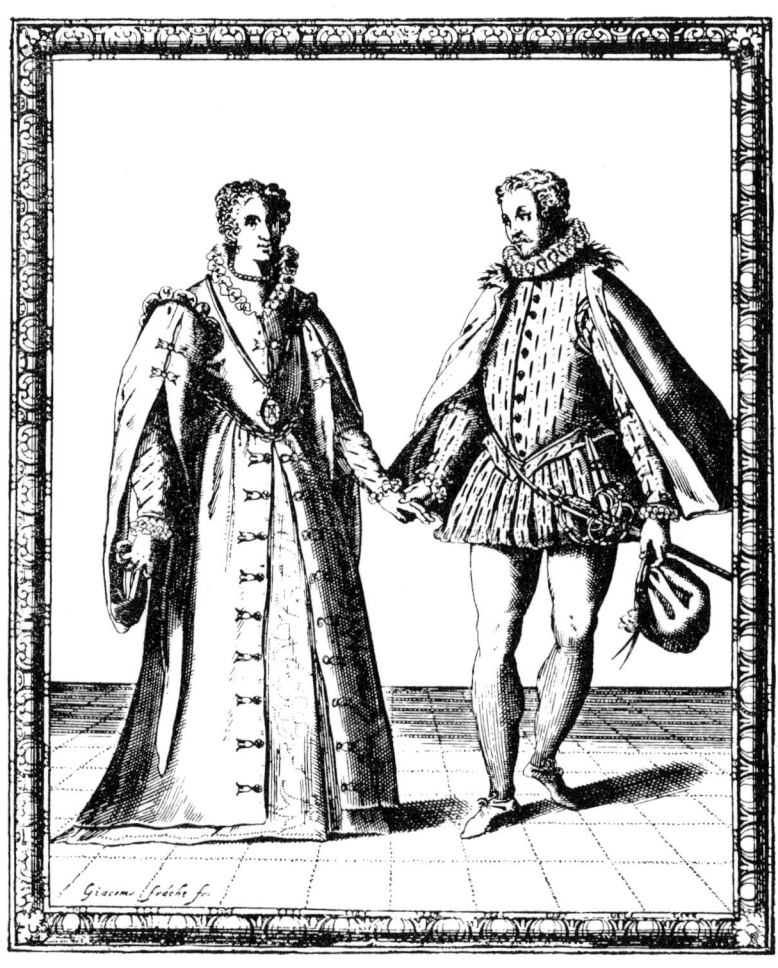

(*From 'Il Ballarino' by Fabritio Caroso*)

BEHAVIOUR AND DEPORTMENT IN THE BALLROOM

FOR LADIES OR GENTLEMEN to appear in the ballroom in the sixteenth century, it was not thought enough to be accomplished dancers. They had to know and observe the rules and conventions of polite society as well; and these, more strict than they are now, gave a particular character to their dancing, so that a little detailed description will help towards a better understanding of the style of their dances. It must be borne in mind that dignity and courtliness were considered social graces, and, while these should be cultivated, a pompous manner and affected gestures, should not be mistaken for them; and, at the same time, a single modern gesture or expression shows itself to be false immediately.

At formal functions, the ladies remained seated while the gentlemen stood, and if a gentleman wished to ask a lady to honour him in the dance, he made his bow with the left foot, taking his hat off with the left hand. In taking it off and putting it on again, he had to be careful to turn the inside down and away from the lady, so that she should not see the moisture gathered by his exertions on the lining. As Caroso remarks with homely insight, 'everyone cannot wear a new hat every day'. The lady then offered her hand and allowed herself to be led to where the dancing was to begin. The gentleman held her hand a little above waist height allowing it to rest lightly in his without grasping it too tightly. As he was expected to wear his cloak, he wrapped it round his left arm, if it was long enough, as it usually was; and, with his hand he held the pommel of his sword, so that the point was turned slightly forward out of harm's way. If he was not wearing a sword, he rested his left hand on his hip, with the knuckles on the hip and the palm turned backwards.

When the lady was asked to dance, she bowed, while remaining seated, and then gave her left hand to the gentleman; but on returning to her seat after the dance, she bowed to the person seated on her right, and, having swept her train under the chair with a slight movement of her body to the left, she seated herself and bowed to the person on the other side. The correct way was to stand a little way from the chair, and then sit down in the middle of the seat, by which means the farthingale was made to fold up and the dress fall to the ground in straight folds. If she was so careless and inexperienced as to sit on the edge of the chair and slide herself back into it, her farthingale rose up and her legs were exposed to view. Farthingales being made of whalebone in those days, they were not so flexible as the steel hoops we use now, but even these need careful management to make them swing and fold up in the right way.

When the various couples had taken their places in readiness for the dance to begin, the musicians usually played the first two bars of the music, to allow them to make the bow; or, if the phrasing of the music did not allow of this, the musicians played a broken chord or arpeggio, which they sustained for the same length of time as the two bars. In set dances, the bow had its own place at the beginning of the strain, and fitted in with the succeeding steps. In the case of the dances that are dealt with in this book, the bow comes outside the actual dance.

If the dance was not vocal, conversation was permitted for those who felt themselves able to dance and talk at the same time; but one imagines that this practice was deprecated by serious dancers, as much then as now. There were not very many dances where conversation was really possible, however proficient the dancers might be, and the Pavan, being a quiet, staid sort of dance, was one of the few where it was at all possible to be social at the same time. Sometimes the musicians would pause after several strains, to allow the dancers to converse at their ease before continuing the dance. This is a small point, but one worth noting as having possibilities for dramatic effect.

The general tendency in stage dancing to-day is for all movements to be large and spacious; in those days, neatness and precision were the ideals, and the modern dancer should be careful to keep his steps and movements controlled. The Italian dancing masters used finger-lengths and hand-breadths to measure the size of steps, and, although Arbeau never gives actual measurements like these in his descriptions, he does state that 'care should be taken that you do not take such long steps that it would seem as if you wished to measure the length of the room, since the damsel cannot in modesty take such long paces as you can'.

The following quotation from the *Memorandum Book of J. Paggitt* (1632-3) is useful as showing very clearly the style that was most admired and cultivated.

'I. ffollow your daucing hard till you have gott a habit of dauncing neately.

II. Care not to daunce loftily, as to carry your body sweetly and smoothly away with a graceful comportment.

III. In some places hanging steps are very graceful and withal give you much ease and time to breath.

IV. Write the marks for the stepps in every daunce under the notes of the tune, as the words are in songs.'

THE BOW OR REVERENCE

THERE appears to have been a diversity of opinion as to which foot the bow was to be made with, but it seems clear that in France they made it with the right foot, in Provence with the left foot and in Italy with whichever foot they fancied. In any case, the movement was the same, the only difference in bows being their duration. The Italians had three kinds: the first which they called Riverenza Grave, occupied the time of four semibreves, the second which they called Riverenza Minima, the time of two semibreves; and the third called Mezza Riverenza occupied the time of one semibreve. The difference between this last bow and the other two was that it never came at the beginning of a dance, as the others did, but was used as a step in passing in the course of a dance.

Supposing the bow (Riverenza Grave) to be done with the left foot, it is executed in the following manner:

Standing with the left foot a little in advance of the right, point the toe of the left foot, and draw it back so that the foot flattens on to the ground as it passes the heel of the right foot, and, taking care to keep it flat, slide it to a position about nine inches behind the right foot. The legs should be kept straight until the left foot is level with the right foot, and, as it passes to the back, incline the body and head a little forwards, and bend both knees, allowing the weight to fall slightly on to the left leg. Then close the left foot against the right, straightening the body and the knees, rising on to the toes as the feet close and then lowering the heels. During the course of this movement the hat is taken off, swept downwards and outwards, and held against the thigh, as has been described; and replaced only on rising from the inclined position.

The lady's bow is the same, except that she does not incline her body as she bends her knees, and, having no hat to take off, she simply opens her hands with the palms turned outwards and lets them fall again as she rises.

THE PAVAN
HISTORY

THE PAVAN is a stately processional dance and depends upon the simultaneous swaying movement and the rise and fall of a large company of dancers for its full effect. Thoinot Arbeau, in his *Orchesographie* (Langres 1588), writes: 'And as for the Pavane, it is used by Kings, Princes and great Lords, to display themselves on some day of solemn festival, with their fine mantles and robes of ceremony and then the Queens and the Princesses, and the Great Ladies accompany them with the long trains of their dresses let down and trailing behind them, or sometimes carried by damsels. These Pavanes, played by hautboys and sackbuts, are called the Grand Bal, and last until those who dance have circled two or three times round the room, if they do not prefer to dance by advances and retreats. These Pavanes are also used in a masquerade, when there is a procession of triumphal chariots of gods and goddesses, emperors or kings resplendent with majesty.'

The Pavan was danced at the courts of Henry VIII and Francis I, and at the numerous Italian courts during the first half of the sixteenth century; and, although it fell out of favour with the French and the Italians, it was still danced at Queen Elizabeth's court right to the end of the century and on into the reign of James I.

The Italians called it Pavana or Paduana, the French called it Pavane, which is the most well-known variation of the word; in England they called it Pavin mostly, and sometimes even Pavine, with that characteristic aptitude for perverting foreign words that they seem to have had even in those days. The reason why the dance is so named is still a matter of doubt. A favourite and picturesque theory is that it was so named from a fancied resemblance to the strut of a peacock, but some observation of a peacock in motion leads one to the conclusion that it must have been a poor sort of compliment to the dancer, the peacock having little grace or dignity that might serve as a model. A certain air of dignity is lent to the peacock by its brilliant and extensive plumage. It is true that the word *pavoneggiare* occurs in descriptions of steps and movements by contemporary dancing masters, and this may be translated as meaning 'to peacock', or in other words, to move in the supposed manner of a peacock. As this term appears in the descriptions of a number of different dances, these might all have been named Pavana with equal justice. Another explanation is that the name came from the town of Padua, where it was first danced. This seems a more likely explanation, as it was quite a usual custom in those days to name a dance after its place of origin.

THE PAVAN—HISTORY

The Pavan must have come into fashion in the beginning of the century, as the first known music is to be found in a collection called *Intabolatura De Lauto*, by Petrucci (Venice, 1508); presumably the dance came into being a little earlier than this. It is significant that the dance is here named Padoana. In all probability, some kind of processional parading being already in use, it became simplified and fixed in a definite form about this time.

In the early sixteenth century, Italy and the Netherlands were foremost in the cultivation of the Arts, and the spirit of the Renaissance was finding its highest expression through the minds of Leonardo da Vinci, Michael Angelo, Erasmus and Castiglione, to name but a few; and the music and movements of the Pavan seem to possess some of the qualities of grandeur and dignity that characterise the work of these great men. At the beginning of the century, the Netherlands vied with Italy where the arts of music and dancing were concerned; but in another fifty years, the Italians were without a rival, and from them springs the great tradition of classical dancing that we have to-day.

The French court was influenced a great deal by the Flemish school on the one side, and the Italian school on the other; and, besides having their own traditional branles, which were the dances of the peasantry, the pavans, galliards and corantos were much in vogue. The Provençal school, about which mention has already been made, was really separate from the rest of France, having had a culture of its own dating back more than a hundred and fifty years, from the time when the Popes were in exile at Avignon. Antonius d'Arena, the Provençal poet and lawyer, is the chief authority for their manner of dancing. His book *Ad Suos Compagnognes* . . . (1536), although written in macaronic verse and difficult to elucidate, is of great value with regard to the dances of the early part of the century.

The Italians were not much influenced by the French style of dancing, although the term *alla Francese* is found occasionally in some of the Italian books on dancing in the latter part of the century.

The English seem to have had very few, if any, court dances of their own, being too busy always with civil wars and fighting with other countries; and the Pavan, the Galliard and the Coranto were all imported from abroad. These began to become more popular among the upper classes after the meeting of Henry VIII and Francis I on the 'Field of the Cloth of Gold', and everything that was French took the English fancy, as it seems to have done ever since. The Flemish 'Bassedanses' found their way to England some time during these years, and the Italian ambassadors, with their numerous attendant gentlemen and servants, did a great deal towards popularising their own dances at the English court. A little treatise entitled *The Manner to Dance Basse Dances*, which was published in 1521, is the first known book on dancing ever to be produced in England. Although of slight value for the information it gives on its subject, it points to an increasing interest in the more sophisticated and complex developments of the art that were taking place on the Continent. The type of dance known as 'bassedanse', was going out of fashion in the French and Italian courts, and the Pavan, which is only a simplified bassedanse, retained the character of the older type of dance to a more marked degree than its contemporaries.

As a processional dance, the Pavan was used for the opening of Court balls, when the older people could dance sedately, and everyone was glad of the opportunity for showing off their rich clothes. Sometimes they sang as they danced, a custom more common in the previous century than in the sixteenth, and rapidly dying out, although popular songs were often used as the basis for dance tunes well into the seventeenth century. Arbeau gives an example of a vocal Pavan in 2/4 time beginning *Belle qui Tiens Ma Vie*. It is the only one written out in four-part harmony, and, as it is easily accessible in C. Beaumont's translation of the *Orchesographie*, it has not been included among the examples at the end of this book.

The Italians invented a variation on the Pavan which they called Passa-mezzo, in English, 'half-step' and, whereas the Pavan was almost always written in common time, the Passa-mezzo was written in 2/4 time and the dancers executed twice as many steps to a beat as in the Pavan, which explains the name of the dance. The whole character of the dance was lively, and it was probably invented to please the younger people who demanded something less solemn to follow, or to dance instead of the Pavan.

In Spain, the Spanish Pavan or Pavaniglia was the equivalent of the Passa-mezzo, and Caroso gives an example in *Il Ballarino*, with a tune by Antonio Cabeçon, the blind Spanish composer, that was popular all over Europe. Music for the Passa-mezzo appears for the first time in *Intabolatura Del Lauto*, by Antonio Rotta (1546), and it gradually superseded the Pavan, until by the middle of the century, the latter is no longer heard of in Italy. In France and England it still continued, and the musical form was used by the great Elizabethan composers as a vehicle for compositions of the highest order. It will be understood that many of these pieces were not intended to be used for dancing, and those that were are identifiable by a steady rhythmic beat running through the music, unbroken by the complex embroideries that otherwise distinguish the viol fantasies and other instrumental pieces. The Passa-mezzo appears in the early seventeenth century, when a new type of dancing was gradually coming into fashion.

MUSIC

THE MUSIC for the Pavan was usually written in common time, as has already been noted, and, in England it was customary to divide the tune into three strains of eight, twelve and sometimes sixteen bars, each of which was repeated once. The continental composers did not keep to such strict form, but made their music according to their own fancy, only observing the rule that, however many strains they made, these had to be phrased in sets of four bars as the arrangement of the steps demanded. Thomas Morley writes in his *Plaine and Easy Introduction to Practical Musicke* (1594) '... if you keep to that rule it is no matter how many foures you put in your straine, for it will fall out well enough in the ende'.

As regards the playing of the music, an orchestra composed of strings, and a harpsichord, is the ideal. This may be supplemented with advantage, by oboes, recorders, or possibly, flutes, if recorders are not available; and, of course, a drum, which is essential for this type of dance music, however small the orchestra may be. Where a large orchestra is not possible, a small one with a virginals and a drum, are adequate for small productions. A piano should be used as a last resort. The atmosphere conveyed by the thickened tones of this instrument is entirely foreign to the spirit of the music.

THE STEPS

THE STEPS used in dancing the Pavan are few in number, and appear simpler than they really are. They consist entirely of two *singles* and one *double*, the sequence being repeated indefinitely, beginning first with one and then the other foot.

A *single* is a plain walking step forward, the back foot following after it has moved; each single step is equal in time to one semibreve; therefore two are equal to one bar of music. The step may also be done backwards.

A *double* is three walking steps forwards, closing the back foot to the one in front after the third step, and each double is equal in time to two semibreves; therefore, one double is equal to one bar of music. The sequence may be done backwards also and in other dances it is done to the side.

HISTORICAL DANCES FOR THE THEATRE

The first *single* is made with the left foot, the second with the right foot and the *double* begins with the left. The whole sequence is then begun again with the right foot, and as each sequence occupies four bars of music, it will be understood why Thomas Morley insisted that the music should be made in sets of fours.

The above description gives the plain steps, only without the bends and rises that turn them from mere marching steps into dancing ones. To do it with style and grace, these must be fully understood.

When the *single* is made to the left, bend the knees and curve the body (*pavoneggiare*) towards the left side and step a little to the side as well as forwards, rising on to the toes as the right foot is brought up. Lower the heels and bend the knees as the next movement with the right foot is made. The *single* with the right foot is made in the same way.

When the *double* is made, the first step is done with a bend, the second on the toes, and the third with a bend and curve of the body as the other foot is brought up to it, remembering always to rise on the toes as the feet are closed together, and to lower the heels *only* as the next step is made. In this way, the swaying motion of the whole company of dancers is made possible. The *double* should be made going forward and not to the side as the *singles* are done.

The Italians sometimes made their *singles* and *doubles* without bringing the feet together, and in Provence they sometimes made three movements of the *single* and five of the *double*, in this way; after the first step of the *single* to the left, the right foot is quickly brought up to it and the left is advanced again; this is repeated with the right foot; and in doing the *double*, two plain steps are taken and then three quicker ones, as in the single. To fit these extra steps into the same time it is necessary to dance them at a livelier speed; and so a more lilting rhythm than the other comes about. This type of step is more suited to the Pavan in 3/4 time, and is nearer in style to the Passa-mezzo. Arbeau registers his disapproval of the step, but, as the recognised Provençal style, there is no reason why it should not be employed when the occasion requires it.

THE FIGURES

THE PAVAN is usually danced by couples in a column going clockwise round the room, with the gentlemen on the outside. Sometimes it is danced by advances and retreats, and sometimes the dancers lead up the middle of the room, separate, and cast off to the bottom of the room, coming up the middle again. Without doing violence to the traditional figures, others may be devised, but these should always be in fairly strict formation, and bows should not be introduced again after the first one, until the very end of the dance.

THE MINUET

Part One: History

THE GENERAL NATURE OF THE MINUET

LIKE many another good dance before and since, the Minuet fell upon a period of disuse. But because it was a famous product of an exceptionally brilliant age, it has been remembered in name, and pressed into service in a long series of historical plays, pageants and fancy-dress balls. It must be realised quite clearly that these survivals do not bear much relation to the true nature of the Minuet. With the possible exception of the Pavan and the Gavotte, the Minuet has suffered more from foolish renderings than any other dance. Audiences of to-day are so used to seeing ladies and gentlemen in powdered wigs and lace, mincing round one another with curtsies, smiles and hand-kissings, that they may well be pardoned for dismissing the Minuet as an affected and somewhat ridiculous affair, of little interest to-day, save to the lovers of the 'quaint' and 'old-fashioned'.

It is not always realised that the Minuet remained in fashion for a period of considerably over a hundred years. The manners and modes of 1650 differed very greatly from those of 1750, but at no time throughout the life of the Minuet is there the slightest suggestion that gentlemen led their ladies through archways of hands, curtseyed, flirted, or ogled, in the course of the dance. P. Rameau, one of the chief authorities on the Minuet, lays especial emphasis on the need to avoid all affectation. He desires the dancers to preserve a calm bearing and an air of natural dignity. A very little experience will serve to show that a curtsey introduced into the middle of a dance would spoil the smooth gliding effect proper to the style, and would effectively destroy the dignity of the general impression. Like 'pump-handling' in a Mayfair ballroom of to-day, it would have been regarded as a grave lapse of taste. The dance is sufficiently beautiful without the addition of unwanted airs and graces.

To what are we to attribute these mistaken versions of the Minuet? It is possible that many errors can be traced to a number of contemporary pictures, somewhat misleading to those whose ideas of the dance were already not very clear. There is a well-known engraving, reproduced in Cecil Sharp's book *The Dance*, called *Le Bal Paré*. It shows a dance in progress which might be taken for a Minuet by the uninitiated. But no figure of the kind which the four couples are shown performing has ever found its way into the descriptions of the dancing masters of the time. The *Traité sur l'art de la Danse* of Malpied, which appeared not more than three years previous to the publication of the print, contains no hint of it. A little further study shows that it is quite certainly not part of a Minuet at all, but of a Contredanse of the type that was at that time (1773) popular at the French Court.

It is, moreover, always dangerous to rely too implicitly upon pictorial evidence unless the picture has been drawn for descriptive purposes, as part of an explanatory work upon the subject in question. The artist has to think of too many factors of importance in making his picture a work of art to be able to give his attention to matters of accurate positions and correct grouping. His world is one of the imagination, and not always of the literal fact. To give a relevant example, Watteau's exquisite pictures are of doubtful value as dependable information upon the dances of his day. His period, like his costumes, is of no time but that of his own fancy, and the little dancers that he so frequently introduces into his groups, are performing a dance of his own imagining. Their style and deportment are of the time of Louis XIV and XV, but what they are dancing no one can say. A *Fête Champêtre* in the National Gallery of Scotland, and *The Ball under the Colonnade*, are examples that will make our meaning clear. One of the best representations of a dance of the stately Louis XIV tradition is to be found in the picture known as *Charles II Dancing at a Ball at the Hague*. Since this Ball must have taken place when Charles II was in exile, and before his restoration in 1660, it falls somewhat early in our period. There can be very little doubt that the dance in progress is either the Minuet or the Courante, and it shows the style which was to form the model for many years to come.

Naturally, however, the most authentic pictorial illustrations of any dance, are to be looked for in contemporary books on the art of dancing. Rameau's book *Maître à Danser* (1725), contains numerous pictures of the utmost value, and more particularly in respect of the Minuet, which he describes in great, if involved, detail. His drawings are naive, but very clear. Kellom Tomlinson, an English dancing master and a contemporary of Rameau, gives a picture with each separate figure of the dance, in his book *The Art of Dancing Explain'd* (1735). The standard of draughtsmanship is, incidentally, higher than that of Rameau's, but not more explicit.

The Minuet is a noble and expressive dance, and it deserved its long reign as queen of ballroom dances. It is not easy, however, to understand quite why it should have been singled out for especial preference from among a host of other dances, all equally beautiful, unless it was because, unlike those other dances, it progressed by means of only one basic step, through a series of pre-ordained figures not subject to alteration. In its earlier forms, many types of step were introduced, and a considerable variety of figures; it occurred, moreover, in suites of dances, and the performers were expected to be proficient also in the Courante, the Rigaudon and the Sarabande. In the later period, the Minuet acquired a comparative simplicity of form. Such ornamental variations of the basic step as were retained were optional and, no doubt, the average dancer, as in our own times, would find the minimum equipment sufficient to see him through the dance more or less creditably. The figures of the dance became fixed in an understood form and order, and we rather suspect that the ladies and gentlemen of the Court were beginning to find it easier to accept a stereotyped dance, of which they could be quite sure, than to go to the trouble of taking regular dancing lessons and practising the great variety of steps required to make it possible for them to perform the other contemporary Court dances.

ORIGINS

THE BEGINNINGS of most famous dances are usually obscure. This is true of some popular dances of quite recent origin, and it is still more true when it is necessary to look back into the past through the mist of nearly three hundred years. Much ink could be wasted to little purpose on such questions. It is, after all, a comparatively unimportant matter where a dance came from, or how it was evolved, so long as the freshness and beauty have been preserved and can still give pleasure to the performers and the spectators. But in order to give a clear idea of the nature of the Minuet, it will perhaps, be as well to begin at the beginning, in so far as that can be attempted with any certainty in the case of an art, the first primitive movements of which we are never likely to be able to trace.

There are various suggestions as to the ancestry of the Minuet, and the most favoured is that it was evolved from the Branle de Poitou, a peasant round dance described by Arbeau. Michel Praetorius, in his book *Terpsichore* (Wolfenbüttel, 1612) was the first person to advance this theory. Unfortunately his work contains a great deal of information regarding the French dances which has already been found to be erroneous, and, as he was mis-informed on so many other points, it is reasonable to suppose that he might be mis-informed on this one; and, to say the least of it, the Branle de Poitou bears very little, if any, resemblance to the Minuet. Rameau repeats the theory with the additional information that the adaptation was made by Beauchamp, who was dancing master to Louis XIV. It is possible that Rameau obtained his information from Beauchamp himself, and if this could be proved to have been the case, there would be no further occasion for discussion, but, in the absence of any such proof, there remains the considerable possibility of Rameau being mis-informed. The explanation appears almost too remote to be possible, and there is an alternative which seems more probable. It is more likely that the Minuet was evolved, not from the rural Branle de Poitou, but from the more sophisticated Galliard, the most popular of all dances in France and England throughout the greater part of the sixteenth century and the earlier decades of the seventeenth century. The points of resemblance between the Galliard and the Minuet are interesting. The Galliard is a dance in triple time, the steps of which occupy two complete bars of music. It was danced by two people only, as not more than one couple could take the floor at the same time, owing to the nature of the dance. It was begun with a ceremonial bow termed 'honours', the dancers meeting and then separating to opposite ends of the room, passing and re-passing one another a number of times during the course of the dance, concluding with honours. In all these respects, the Minuet is the exact counterpart of the Galliard. Furthermore, the relative position of the Galliard in the due order of the Court Balls, corresponds closely with that held by the Minuet during the later period. During the sixteenth century, a Ball was opened with the Pavan, the dignified processional dance in which everyone joined. The more lively and exacting Galliard, in which the less agile dancers were not accustomed to take part, then followed. In the seventeenth century, the opening dance became the Branle, and the Galliard gave place at first to the Courante, and a little later to the Minuet. The connection between the Galliard and the Minuet seems a reasonable inference from these pieces of evidence.*

---

* Regarding the theory that the Galliard is the original source from which the Minuet was adapted and not the Branle de Poitou.

The author is well aware that this theory may arouse controversy, but feels that it is more justified than the others; the Branle de Poitou does not appear to have any single point of resemblance to the Minuet, if the description given in Thoinot Arbeau's *Orchesographie* (1588) is to be relied upon. Mrs. Arnold Dolmetsch, who is well-known as an authority on the dances of the past, is in agreement with the author regarding this matter.

HISTORICAL DANCES FOR THE THEATRE

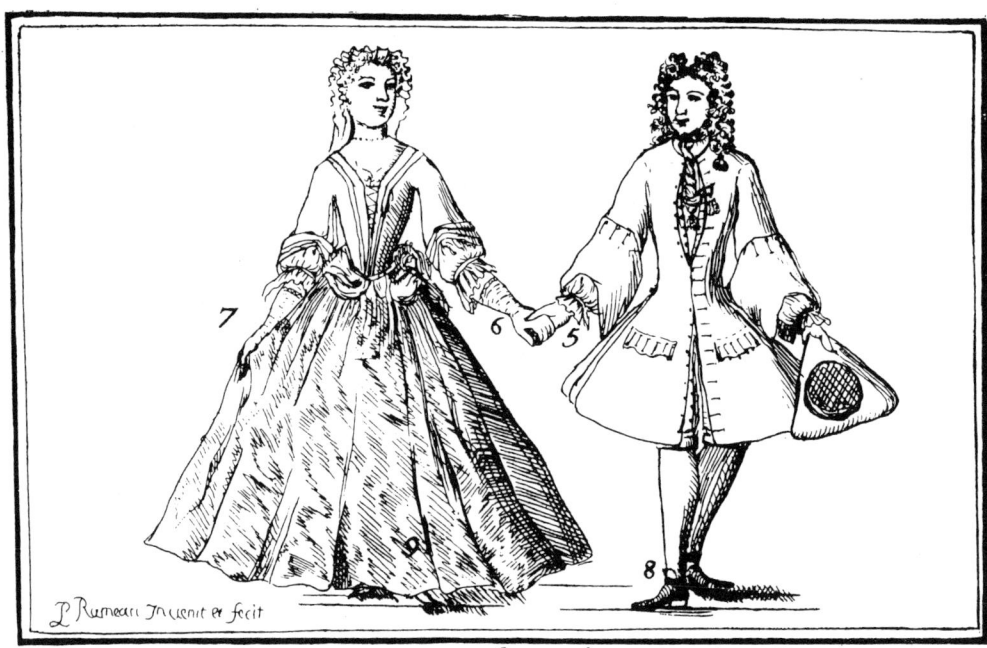

Homme et Femme prest a faire la premier Reverence avant de Dancer

(This plate and those appearing on pp. 31, 36, 38, 40, 41, 43, 45, 46, 47 are from 'Le Maître à Danser' by P. Rameau)

THE MINUET—ORIGINS

As Maître de Ballet to the Court, Beauchamp would make it a part of his business to invent new *enchainements* and new figures for each successive ballet created by himself and the composer Lully, for the entertainment of Louis XIV and his *entourage*. It is not difficult to see how the Galliard, having already acquired a stateliness more in conformity with the tastes of the mid-seventeenth century than it originally possessed, might lend itself to transformation into a new form, as pleasing for the beauty of Lully's music as for the subtle dignity of the new dance itself.

Louis XIV was an excellent dancer, if we may believe the words of contemporary writers. At any rate, he was a very active one, for we are given to understand that Beauchamp gave him a lesson every day as long as he continued to dance. The Courante was his favourite dance, and was for this reason placed first in order of precedence after the ceremonial opening of the *Grand Bal*, until its ultimate displacement by the Minuet. Beauchamp himself partnered the King in a Minuet in the ballet entitled *Le Triumphe de l'Amour*. It appears probable that a number of similar occasions introduced the Minuet to public favour before it took its place as a popular ballroom dance.

The most rigid rules were observed in the conduct of the *Grandes Bals* of Louis XIV. Each dance came in a pre-arranged order. First of all everyone assembled; the King, the Queen, and the members of the Royal family remaining seated. When the King rose, as a sign that the Ball was to begin, everyone present did likewise. The King and the Queen took up their positions at the top of the room, near the musicians, and the Royal Family and the Court arranged themselves in order of precedence behind. The ladies stood to the right and the gentlemen to the left. The processional Branle was then danced, followed by the Gavottes in the same order of couples. It should be remembered here that the Gavottes were not the affected affairs seen in pantomimes to-day. They were actually a collection of round dances known as Branles, and not one single dance. The couples then returned to their places, after bowing to the Presence and also to one another. At this stage came the *Dances a deux*: in other words, the Minuets. I will not presume to improve on Rameau's words, since his description of the procedure is as clear as could be wished, and I therefore give them here: '. . . when the King has danced the first Minuet, he goes to his seat and everyone sits down, for, while His Majesty is dancing, all stand. Then the Prince who is to dance next after His Majesty is seated, makes him a very profound bow, and then goes to the Queen or the first Princess of the Blood, and together they make the same bows as before the dance. Afterwards they dance the Minuet, and, at the conclusion, make the same bows again. Then the Lord makes a very low bow to the Princess on leaving her, because she will not appear again before the King. At the same time, he advances three or four steps forwards, to salute with another bow the Princess or Lady whose turn is next, to invite her to dance with him. Then he awaits her, so that together they may make a low bow to the King, as shown by these numbers 1, 2 (*a*)* when they descend a little lower, according to the numbers 3, 4 (*b*) and make the customary bows before dancing, and perform the Minuet. At the end of this dance they make the usual bows. Finally, on leaving her, he makes a bow backwards and returns to his place; when the Lady observes the same ceremonial to invite another Prince, and so on to the end.

But if His Majesty desire another dance to be performed, one of the First Gentlemen of the Bedchamber announces his wish, which does not prevent the same bows being observed.' (*c*)

The mode of procedure described in this quotation corresponds to that known at an earlier date, and in connection with the Galliard, *à la Lyonnaise*. Rameau then explains how at all well-regulated Assemblies outside the Court itself, a King and Queen were chosen from among those present, and the same etiquette was observed as though they had been of Royal Blood. It should be remembered that although he was writing in 1725, some seventy years after the first introduction of the Minuet, Rameau was describing an order of procedure which held favour over a long period of years, not only in France, but throughout the Courts of Europe, with few modifications.

The Minuet was first introduced into England, at the Court of Charles II, by the Marquis de Flamarens, whose sole claim to distinction this would appear to have been, since, according to the Marquis de Grammont, he was neither good looking nor witty. Since the Courante was the favoured dance of the moment, it is probable that the Minuet did not at once become universally popular in this country. Charles II never cared for it as much as did Louis XIV. He was not so good a dancer, and perhaps he could not perform it with the necessary ease and grace. His preference was for the Passepied, or 'Paspy', as Pepys called it. The Passepied is the same dance as the Minuet, in essentials, but it is taken in quicker time and

---

* Regarding the numbers in the text where the quotation from Rameau occurs.
These numbers 1, 2, 3 and 4 refer to the position of the dancers in the engraving given in Rameau's *Maître a Danser*, which shows the ballroom with a Ball in progress. 1 and 2 show the Lady and Gentleman bowing to the King, and 3 and 4 show the same Lady and Gentleman, having bowed to the King and each other, in the position at the bottom of the room ready to begin their Minuet.

for this reason it is somewhat easier to perform. Slow movements which call for perfect balance and style, are always more difficult to execute.

The Minuet steps, described later in this book, can be used in performing a Passepied, if they are taken at a quicker speed, and the more complicated ones are omitted.

THE GOLDEN PERIOD

THE FIRST written example of the Minuet known to us appears in Feuillet's *Chorégraphie ou l'Art de Décrire La Dance par Caractères, Figures et Signes Demonstratif*, published in 1701. This book explains the system of notation invented by Beauchamp, by which dances could be recorded in writing and read by dancers, as musicians read music. While this system had its limitations, it also possessed certain advantages, and, above all, was the means of preserving a great number of lovely dances that would otherwise have reached us as names only. Feuillet, having undertaken to write the first book of this kind, acquired the credit—to which he was not entitled—for the invention of the system itself. We are told by P. Siris, in his translation of Feuillet's work published in London in 1706, under the title *The Art of Dancing Demonstrated by Characters and Figures*, that Beauchamp had informed him some years previously that he was the inventor of the system. The point seems to have led to considerable dissension between the two men, but the details of their quarrel do not concern us now. What is important is that such a system should have been invented, no matter by whom, and have been used to record dances in writing for the benefit of posterity. Feuillet's book has given us, by this means, the first known Minuet of which the record has survived. It is the *Menuet et Bourrée a Deux* from the opera *Achille*. The music of part of this work is by Lully; but the composer did not live to complete his score, and only the first Act is from his pen. The Opera was completed by Pascal Colasse: the tune of the *Menuet et Bourree d'Achille* does not appear in the printed version, but since its style proclaims it a probable composition of Lully himself, it is likely that it forms an additional number originally included in a later Act.

The dances for *Achille* are by Louis Pécour, who was Beauchamp's successor as *Maître de Ballet* at the Opera. It is possible that the Minuet in question may have been the work of Beauchamp himself. Pécour is known to have made use, in the early part of his career, of a number of compositions from his master's hand.

At the period with which we are now dealing—the closing years of the seventeenth century and the early part of the eighteenth—it was usual to couple a grave measure with a gay one, to produce an effect of contrast. The Bourrée is a dance in the gay style, which often served as a companion, both to the Minuet and to other stately dances, such as the Chaconne or the Passacaille. Purcell, Lully, and many other contemporary composers, began to write Minuets, not only for dancing, but in Suites intended for instrumentalists alone. The operas and ballets of Lully are inexhaustible storehouses of lovely dance tunes, not least of Minuets; and up to the close of the eighteenth century, great composers continued to add to their number. With the choice of such composers as Rameau, Handel, Haydn and Mozart before them, it is difficult to understand why modern choreographers should cling so tenaciously to the superficialities of a Boccherini or a Gretry, as though such composers formed the only source of Minuets, good or bad. In truth, the available supply of Minuet movements is very rich and varied.

The English translation of 1706 by P. Siris, of Feuillet's books, was preceded by another translation in the same year by John Weaver; that of Siris contained, however, some additional matter. These publications were the signal for a flood of books containing collections of dances, and many Minuets from the contemporary operas appeared in this form, mostly composed for two dancers and sometimes for four. Mr. Isaac, dancing master to the Princess Anne, composed at least one solo Minuet for the Princess herself. Kellom Tomlinson also composed Minuets for two, incorporated in Suites which contained, in addition, Entrees, Rigaudons and Passepieds.

The Minuet had now reached the height of its fashion.

But at this point it becomes necessary to draw a distinction (when dealing with its development) between the two forms of the dance which by this time had become more apparent: the Minuet of the Ballet or Opera, and that of the ballroom, where its popularity was to become so great and long-lived. The former included a greater variety of steps, and the figures might be devised in accordance with the fancy of the choreographer. The *Menuet et Bouree d'Achille* previously mentioned, the Minuets for four dancers in Gaudrau's collection, and several of those in Tomlinson's collection, may be cited as typical examples of this category; but those of Rameau and others of Tomlinson's, are of the ballroom type. In this form the figures are fixed and invariable, and the dance requires one basic step alone. Other steps might be introduced by the more enterprising and accomplished dancers, but those of average attainments could content themselves, as in the ballroom of to-day, with a minimum of variety and elaboration.

THE MINUET—FURTHER DEVELOPMENTS

The great professional dancers of the late seventeenth and early eighteenth centuries, passed on the principles of their technique and style to pupils who carried on their tradition undiminished. Blondy, Beauchamp's nephew; Marcel, who could sing as well as dance; Ballon, whose grace and lightness were accounted unsurpassable; Mlles. Subligny, Guiot, Prévost, Sallé and Camargo: these were among the great names at the Opera at the time when the Minuet was at the height of its vogue. It is from this, the Golden Period, that we shall select the example used for illustration in the second part of this book.

FURTHER DEVELOPMENTS

AS THE CENTURY progressed, many dances of the Court tradition disappeared from ballroom use; but the Minuet continued in unchallenged supremacy. As Pepys informed us, dances of an entirely different type—the Country Dances—had come into great favour in England at the Court of Charles II. Now, to the great disgust of the older professional dancing masters, and in the face of their not unnatural opposition, the Country Dances succeeded in invading the select circle of Louis XV himself. They underwent, as might be expected, many curious changes in the process. The balancé, the pas de rigaudon, and similar ornamental steps, were grafted on to them by way of variety; and new dances were invented with flowery or classical names and tunes of an excessively languishing type. Throughout all these sophistications the Minuet remained unchanged. Once established in its prescribed figures and steps, it seems to have undergone no serious modification from the time of Rameau and Tomlinson to that of Malpied's *Traité sur l'Art de la Danse*, which appeared about 1770, and which re-affirmed the principles laid down by Feuillet seventy years before. Only one change occurred worth remarking. The main figure was planned as an S by Beauchamp, but had been altered to a Z by Pécour, an innovation which, although regarded as of the greatest importance at the time, no longer seems of much moment to us.

With certain exceptions, the great dancers of the eighteenth century did not concern themselves with the Minuet. Now that the dance had largely passed from the theatre and the professional world into the sphere of the ballroom, their time was too fully engaged with the newest demands upon their technique for them to give much attention to the quieter ballroom types; nevertheless, the exceptions are worth noting. We have already mentioned Ballon, with his reputation for lightness. He was dancing master to the Royal Family and the Court of

Louis XV; his nephew, Bandiery Laval, and the latter's son, Michel Bandiery Laval, filled the same post in succession to one another. Marcel, for many year after he became unable to dance himself, taught deportment and the refinements of the Minuet.

We are told by contemporary writers that he was very strict with his pupils, criticising their shortcomings freely, irrespective of rank.

Mlle. Camargo, of whom there is a beautiful painting by Lancret in the Wallace Collection, was one of the most celebrated dancers of this, or any century; her grace in dancing the Minuet is said to have been unsurpassable, and her interpretation of both the Minuet and the Passepied was thought to excel that of Mme. Prevost, whose pupil she was, because she was more 'turned out' than her teacher.

In England, Tomlinson was teaching the aristocracy how to dance and how to carry themselves in the ballroom, at a guinea and a half for twelve lessons; and Beau Nash, who died in 1762, upheld for half a century the traditions of politeness and good breeding in the Assembly Room at Bath. It was Beau Nash who compelled the men to leave their swords at home when they came to the Assembly, and who made them wear shoes instead of boots when dancing, considering quite rightly, that to dance the Minuet gracefully in boots was not really possible. We find Thomas Wilson still emphasising the same necessity as late as 1816.

Throughout the latter half of the eighteenth century the Minuet remained the first dance at Balls and Court functions, and, indeed, at every Assembly in Europe where there was dancing. Although some small variations in the step occurred, the figures were invariably the same. The little ornamental French Contre-danses, danced in sets for as many as would, continued to attract popular fancy, and the vogue for Country Dances continued unabated in England. About 1770, the Quadrille, which had recently come into fashion in France, was transported into England, where it rapidly grew in popularity. The day of the Minuet was over. Its decline coincided with the end of an historical period; in some degree, perhaps, it symbolised the typical characteristics of its time. The French Revolution effectively put an end to it in France, and, since France set the fashion in dancing as well as in dressing at that time, as now, fashionable society in the European capitals followed suit, and Quadrilles, Cotillons, and Country Dances soon became universally popular. In England it was still the custom to open a Ball with the Minuet in the first decades of the nineteenth century, but we read in *A Treatise on Dancing*, published at Norwich in 1820, that it was then only danced at Court Balls and had fallen out of fashion elsewhere.

THE MINUET—FURTHER DEVELOPMENTS

Princess Victoria danced the Minuet at various social functions when she was still a child, but it is not mentioned as ever having been danced at Buckingham Palace after she became Queen. Quadrilles, Lancers and Waltzes seem to have completely displaced it, and so the Minuet may be said to have become a relic of the past, having been in vogue for a hundred and fifty years.

THE MINUET
Part Two
HOW TO DANCE THE MINUET

IT IS ASSUMED that the majority of those who wish to learn how to dance the Minuet have a general knowledge of the technical terms used in dancing; that is to say, such points as the five positions of the feet, the five positions of the arms, the seven movements used in dancing and a few other essentials.

Those unacquainted with these definitions may study them in textbooks on the art of classical dancing and, therefore, they will not be described here; but the descriptions of the steps and figures have been made as simple and explicit as possible, so that the lack of this knowledge does not really constitute a serious difficulty.

While, however, the author has tried to explain each step and movement of the dance as clearly as possible, it must be realised that the Feuillet system of dance notation, to which reference has already been made, will convey a far more graphic picture of the dance than any amount of written description, no matter how detailed. I shall therefore give, in addition to the written account, a complete diagram of the dance in this notation, together with a key to the meaning of the signs employed. By supplementing the diagrammatic notation with the written instructions for the timing of the steps and for the arm and body movements, it is hoped that a fairly accurate conception will be conveyed, not only of the dance itself, but the style in which it should be performed.

Music

In selecting suitable music, it is necessary to discriminate between that which was written expressly for dancing and that which was intended for instrumentalists alone. The Minuets in the Suites of Bach are mostly unsuitable for dancing, and are moreover, spoiled as pure music by being played either too fast or too slow in order to adapt them to the requirement of the dancers; and as there is a very large quantity of music of the first quality available, it is quite unnecessary to do this violence to the composer's original intentions. Outstanding examples of suitable music for dancing are to be found in the works of Lully and Purcell, for the early period, and in those of Rameau and Handel, for the later period. The numerous collections of dances in notation also provide a rich storehouse of beautiful tunes, which, although rarely found in modern reprints, are easily accessible in the Reading Room of the British Museum.

Tempo

The tempo of the dance must naturally be considered at the same time as the choice of music because of the different speeds at which it was performed during the various stages of its development. It is not generally realised that the Minuet began its career as a comparatively lively dance and in course of time, became slower and more dignified. We find the Abbé Brossard writing in 1703: '. . . One ought, in imitation of the Italians, to use the signature 3/8 or 6/8 to mark its movement, which is always very gay and very fast. But the custom of marking it by a simple 3 or 3/4 has prevailed.' In contrast to this it was possible for Diderot and d'Alembert to write in their *Encyclopédie*, about 1750, that '. . . The character of the Menuet is a noble and elegant simplicity; the movement is moderate rather than quick. It may be said that the least gay of all the kinds of dances used in our balls is the Menuet.' It will be seen then that it is very important to decide whether the earlier or later form of the dance is to be represented. In dancing Minuets from the period included between 1650 and 1710, the dance may be performed at the speed MM. Crochet = 160; from this time onwards it should be taken at about half that speed. This is a fairly safe general rule, but it will be understood that there was no sudden change, and music may be found that seems to require some gaiety in its interpretation and yet belongs to as late a date as 1710. During the nineteenth century it was fashionable to teach a version of the Minuet to young ladies to make them more accomplished, and this was danced at an even slower tempo. As this was a revival and not a continuation of the tradition, it should not be taken as an authoritative precedent.

The Minuet Step

Coming to the minuet step itself, it must be understood first of all, that one minuet step occupies two bars of music. As a result of this, all Minuet tunes written for dancing have an even number of bars in each strain, and, therefore, in a strain of eight bars, the dancers must of necessity execute four minuet steps. To avoid the possibility of confusion between the steps for the first bar and those for the second, we will count these two bars of three beats each as one bar of six beats.

Another important point to be borne in mind, is that every minuet step, no matter in which direction it is taken, must be begun with the right foot. This rule applies whether the step is performed forwards, backwards, turning, or to either side; it is, moreover, still observed with regard to any of the ornamental steps that can be introduced for the sake of variety into the different figures of the dance. When, as is the case in certain of these ornamental steps, the step itself finishes on the right foot, it must be performed twice running in order to allow the next normal minuet step to be taken in the correct manner with the right foot.

We have already mentioned in the preceding chapter that the Minuet was performed in a slightly different manner in England from that of France. Since, therefore, France was the country of its origin, we will begin by describing the way in which it was danced in that country.

The *minuet* step itself consists essentially of four plain steps, beginning with the right foot and ending with the left; these four steps are varied by means of bends and rises, either on or during the beats, and it is the manner in which these bends and rises are disposed that brings about the differences between the French and English versions of the step.

French Style, Forwards

Standing in the third position, left foot front:

BEATS
- ½ Bend the knees.
- 1 Rise and step on to the right foot.
- 2 Bend the knees.
- 3 Rise and step on to the left foot.
- 4 Step on to the right foot without lowering the heels or bending the knees.
- 5 Bend the knees.
- 6 Rise and step on to the left foot.

French Style, Backwards

The same movements as the foregoing are executed in a backward direction, but with this difference, that they are commenced from the first position instead of the third.

French Style, Sideways to the Left

BEATS
- ½ Bend the knees.
- 1 Rise and step to the third position right foot back.
- 2 Bend the knees.
- 3 Rise and step on to the left foot, opening it to the second position.
- 4 Pass the right foot to the third position back without lowering the heel, or bending the knees.
- 5 Bend the knees.
- 6 Rise and step to the second position with the left foot.

If the next *minuet* step is to be done in any other direction, the foot should be brought to the first position instead of the second. There is an alternative way of performing this step to the left, in which the right foot passes in front of the left, the first time it moves, and behind it, the second time. This can have a very charming effect, especially if the dancers make a slight *epaulement* while performing it.

French Style, Sideways to the Right

This is performed in the same manner as the foregoing, except that the right foot opens outwards to the second position from the first, and the left foot passes behind to the third position each time it moves, but, as has already been described, when the succeeding minuet step is to be performed in a different direction, the left foot closes to the first position the last time. The *minuet* step to the right can be made by passing the left foot in front of the right foot the second time it moves. It is sometimes done in this manner when the succeeding minuet step is to be made forwards.

English Style

This style of performing the *minuet* step was known as 'one and a fleuret'; that is, a *demi-coupé*, which is a step with a bend and a rise on it; and a *fleuret*, which is three steps, the first of which has a bend and a rise on it, the other two being pas marches without bends or rises on them. The timing is slightly different from the French step just described.

English Style, Forwards

Standing in the third position right foot back.

BEATS
- ½ Bend the knees.
- 1 Step forward with the right foot.
- 2 Hold the step without bending the knees, but the heel may be lowered.
- 3 Bend the knees.
- 4 Rise and step forward with the left foot.
- 5 Step forward with the right foot on the toes.
- 6 Step forward with the left on the toes.

English Style, Backwards and Sideways

This step is performed in exactly the same way backwards and sideways to the left and right, as has already been described in relation to the French style, using the 'one and a fleuret', and timing the movements in the foregoing manner. The alternative ways of putting the right foot in front the first time it moves when going to the left, and the same in reverse when going to the right, may also be used.

The French and English steps were both used from the first appearance of the Minuet, and were even used together in the same dance, until 1740; but after that date the French step fell out of fashion and the English step was the only one used. Malpied gives only one way of performing it, and that is the English way; he has further complexities and nuances of timing for those occasions when the step is performed sideways and backwards, that do not seem of sufficient importance to need detailed description. Other ways of performing the step are as follows:

The Passepied Step, or the Fleuret and a Bound

This is found in the early Minuets, and both Feuillet and Weaver give it; Rameau and Tomlinson mention it, but the latter says (this is in 1735) that it has fallen out of fashion. The actual sequence consists of a *fleuret* (see English Style, forwards, for definition of a *fleuret*) and a bound. The step is not used continuously, but is only introduced occasionally, or alternated with the other step. It is performed in this way: Standing in the third position right foot back:

BEATS
1. Bend the knees.
2. Rise and step forward on to the right foot.
3. Step forward on to the left foot on the toes.
4. Step forward on to the right foot on the toes.
5. Bend the knees.
6. Bound on to the left foot.

ORNAMENTAL STEPS

The Contretemps

THERE are various other steps of a more or less ornamental nature that may be introduced at appropriate places in the dance, the first and most important of these being the *contretemps*. This consists of a sequence of three movements and is performed in the following manner; standing in the third position right foot back:

BEATS
1. Hop on the left foot, at the same time raising the right foot behind.
2. Pass the right foot forward.

THE MINUET—ORNAMENTAL STEPS

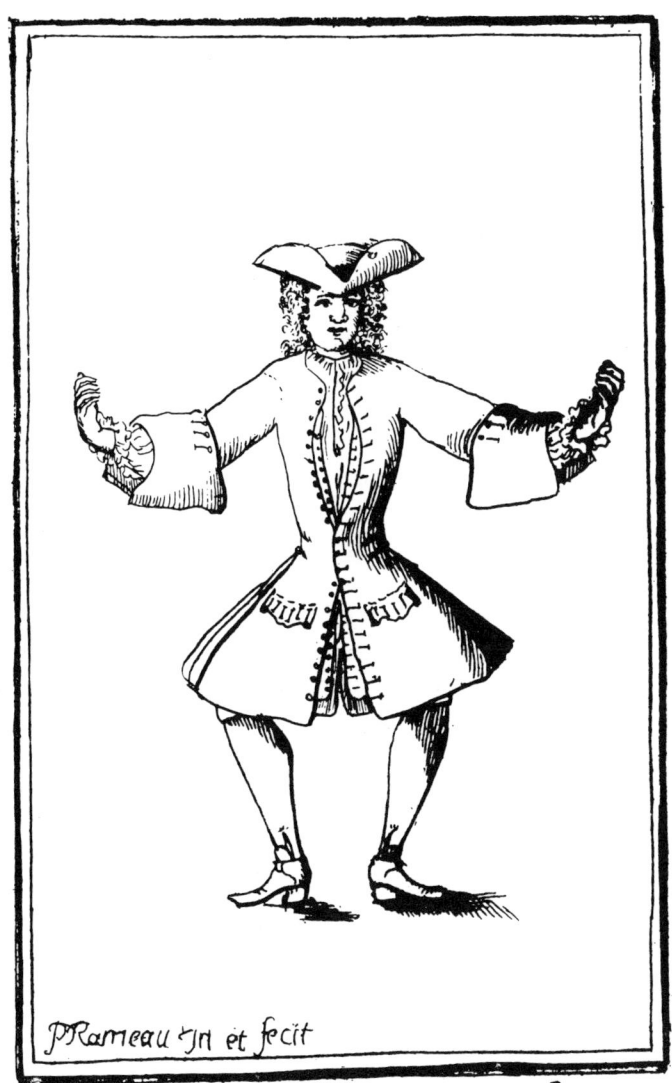

Premier mouvement du
Contretemps

HISTORICAL DANCES FOR THE THEATRE

3   Step on to it.
4   Hop on the right foot and at the same time raise the left foot behind.
5   Close the left foot to the position *sur le cou de pied derrière*.
6   Bound forward on to the left foot.

This step can be performed backwards or turning to the right, and is done in exactly the same way as in going forwards, except that, in executing it backwards, the left foot comes to the position *sur le cou de pied devant* as it closes against the right foot. As a general rule the *contretemps* is not performed twice running in the dance.

The Balancé

This consists of two steps only, one with a bend and a rise, and one with a beat. Like the *contretemps*, it occupies two bars of music and is never executed more than once at a time. It is performed in the following manner: standing in the third position right foot back:

BEATS
1   Bend and rise and step to the second position with the right foot on the toes.
2   *Dégagé* the left foot.
3   Beat the left instep against the right foot, bending the knees at the same time, and lowering the heel of the right foot.
4   Open the left foot to the second position again, straightening the knees, and *dégagé* the right foot.
5, 6   Wait in this position before making the next step.

This step is most appropriate when the succeeding step is to be a *minuet* step to the left, as the right foot may be carried to the third position behind with ease and smoothness, and the first bend can occupy the sixth beat of the *balancé* which remains unused. The *balancé* may also be done forwards. Rameau prefers it so, but it seems equally effective both ways. To do it forwards, step to the fourth position on the first beat, close the left foot to the right heel and back again to the fourth position behind on the third and fourth beats.

The Flying Bourrée

This step consts of three steps, the first one having a bend and a rise on it, and the two succeeding steps being made on the toes. It is performed forwards only in the following manner. Having completed a *minuet* step and the left foot being advanced with the weight on it:

BEATS
1 Bend, rise and step forward with the right foot.
2 Step forward with the left foot on the toes and with the knees straight.
3 Step forward with the right foot on the toe with the knees straight.

This completes the sequence, but as one *flying bourree* occupies only one bar of music, two must be executed in succession to complete the six beats, and to enable the dancer to continue with the *minuet* step. Kellom Tomlinson names it the *flying bourrée*, but in France it was known as the *fleuret*.

The Double Bourrée

This step is seldom used, but is useful to have in reserve if a more sparkling type of Minuet is required. As the name implies, it consists of two *bourrées*, and for this reason; that one would bring the dancer on to the wrong foot for continuing with the *minuet* step. It is performed in this manner. Having completed a *minuet* step with the weight on the left foot:

BEATS
½ Bend and rise.
1 Step to the second position with the right foot and draw the left foot up to the position *sous le cou de pied*, behind, rising on to three-quarter point on the right foot at the same time.
2 Step out to the second position with the left foot.
3 Close the right foot to the third position behind, sliding it in and lowering the heels at the same time.

The step is then repeated in reverse, and a little careful practice is necessary to enable the dancer to execute it smoothly and lightly. The second movement, when the left foot is closed behind the right and then opened, must be balanced with ease, and executed without jerky or unsteady movements.

The Coupée or Marchés

These are two simple steps, each occupying one bar of music and usually performed going forward. They are performed in this manner:

Having completed a *minuet* step and the weight being on the left foot:

BEATS
1 Bend the knees.
2 Slide the right foot forward without lifting the toe off the floor, and rising at the same time.
3 Complete the length of the step.

The step is then repeated with the left foot during the next bar of music, so that, at the completion of it, the weight is off the right foot, leaving it free to begin the *minuet* step which is to follow.

The Slip and Half Coupée

This step is seldom used and, like the *flying bourée* and the *double bourrée*, it must be performed twice, so that the succeeding *minuet* step can begin with the right foot; but, unlike these steps, it occupies two bars of music, or six beats, making four bars in all if the step is done twice. It is performed in this manner. Having completed a *minuet* step and the weight being on the left foot, or with the weight equally distributed and the feet placed in the third position right foot back:

BEATS

1 Bend, rise and step to the second position with right foot.

2-3 Slide the left foot to the third position behind, bending both knees, thus completing the slip.

4 Step forward with the right foot, straightening the knees, thus completing the *coupée*.

5-6 Wait in this position before making the next step.

The step is then repeated in the opposite direction. This completes the whole sequence twice.

THE MINUET STEP AND ORNAMENTAL STEPS LATER PERIOD

ALL THE foregoing steps were employed until about 1750, and it seems that they went out of fashion fairly quickly. Malpied describes only one type of *minuet* step, and this corresponds so nearly to the English *minuet* step that it may be considered the same for all practical purposes. The slight differences of timing when the step is done in different directions, do not seem of sufficient importance to need detailed description. The ornamental steps are of more importance. Malpied gives the *pas grave*, five kinds of *balancés*, one *fleuret* and one rather foolish step which he designates the '*pas de Mons. Marcel*'. We will begin by describing the *pas grave*.

The Pas Grave, Forwards

Standing in the first or third position with the right foot back:

BEATS

1-2
3-4 } Bend, rise and slide the right foot forward to the fourth position.

THE MINUET AND ORNAMENTAL STEPS—LATER PERIOD

5   Close the left foot to the third position back, bending both knees at the same time, but without letting the left foot touch the floor.
6   Rise and step forward on to the left foot.

Pas Grave, Sideways

This step may be done sideways to the right, timing it in exactly the same way as the above. The right foot opens to the second position, and the left foot closes behind it and then passes in front of it to the fourth position across. The step is similar to the *balancé* in construction, but it will be observed that the left foot does not beat against the right, and, after the closed position, the left foot opens forward. The movement must be smooth and unbroken.

The Fleuret

This *fleuret* is remarkably like the *contretemps* of the early period, and is in all probability a modification of the same step. It is performed in the following manner, standing in the first or third position, with the right foot behind:

BEATS
1   Bend, rise and step forward on the right foot.
½   Close the left foot to the third position.
2   Step forward on a bend on to the right foot.
3   Hop on the supporting foot.
4   Close the left foot behind the right without touching the floor, and straighten the right knee.
5   Bend the supporting knee.
6   Bound forward on to the left foot.

The Balancé, Forwards

Of the five ways of performing this step, it is really sufficient to know three, and the most useful of these is the one going forward. It is performed in this manner: standing in the first or the third position, right foot behind:

BEATS
1   Bend, rise and step forward on to the right foot.
2   Stay for this beat in this position.
3   Beat the side of the left foot against the right ankle.
4   Open the left foot to the fourth position back, transferring the weight to it.
5–6 Close the right foot behind the left to the third position with a semi-circular movement.

[35]

HISTORICAL DANCES FOR THE THEATRE

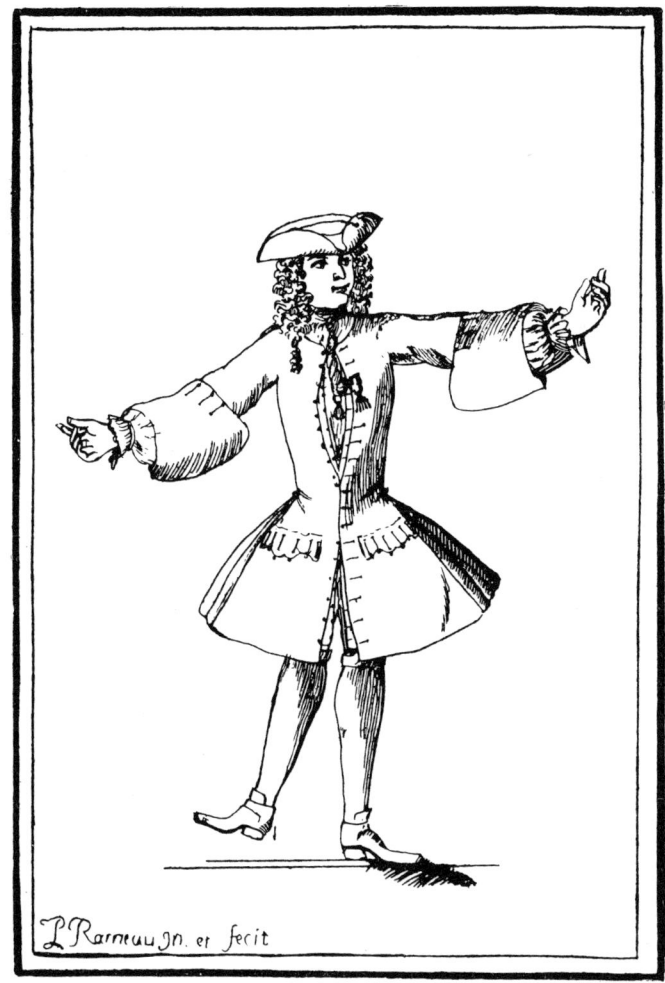

Deuxieme attitude ayant sauté

THE MINUET AND ORNAMENTAL STEPS—LATER PERIOD

If the ensuing step is to be a *minuet* step, it is advisable to put no weight on the right foot as it closes behind the left, so that it will be free to move forward on the next beat.

Balancé, Sideways to the Right

Standing in the first or the third position with the right foot back:

BEATS
1. Bend, rise and step to the second position with the right foot.
2-3. Slide the left foot into the third position back, and bend the knees.
4. Open the left foot to the fourth position back, and straighten the knees.
5-6. Slide the right foot to the first position without putting any weight on it.

Balancé, Turning to the Right

This step can be used in the Z figure instead of the sixth *minuet* step, before moving to the right. It is performed in the following manner: standing in the first position, or the third, with the right foot back:

BEATS
½. Bend the knees.
1-2. Rise, and turning the body a quarter of a turn to the right, step forward on to the right foot.
3-4. Bend, rise and step forward on to the left foot, making a quarter turn to the right, and completing the movement on the fourth beat.
5-6. Raise the right foot and close it behind the left foot with a circular movement, completing the movement on the sixth beat, but without putting any weight on the right foot.

It must be understood that, as the body makes two quarter turns in the course of the balancé, the dancer is then facing the way he came, and the step must be repeated to make a complete turn, so that the *minuet* step which is to follow may continue in the same direction as before. The whole sequence must be executed with perfect balance and smoothness.

Pas de Mons. Marcel

This rather curious step appears to have been invented by Mons. Marcel for his own special purpose, and there is no evidence that it was ever in general use, although one may suppose that he taught it to his own pupils. To execute it, a complete halt is made in the flow of the dance, as it is executed *sur place*. A use might be found for it if the dancers should have to perform in a confined space,

HISTORICAL DANCES FOR THE THEATRE

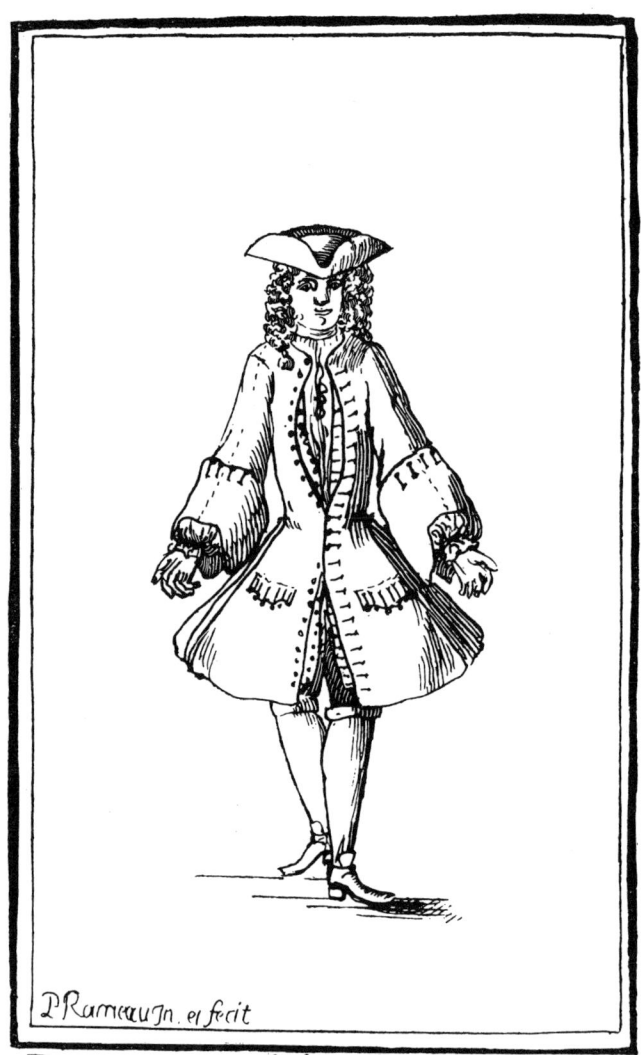

Premiere attitude des bras du Menuet

and for this reason it is included here. Standing in the third position with the right foot in front:

BEATS
1. Bend the knees.
2. Rise on to the toes with a slight spring, changing the position of the feet.
3. Drop back on to the heels, raising the toes off the floor.
4. Raise the heels off the floor.
5. Lower the heels and bend the knees.
6. Execute a small bound on to the left foot, raising the right foot at the back, keeping it close to the supporting foot.

The first movement in this sequence might be called in modern ballet terminology, an *échappé relevé changement*, the two following movements making a kind of rocking motion, and the last movement being simply a bound *sur place*.

Arm movements for the Minuet Step

In performing all *minuet* steps, whether forwards, backwards or sideways, the arm movements are always the same, except in the presenting of hands, which will be described later. For the former, the movements are as follows: at the beginning of the sequence the arms are held in a position that is most accurately described as the fifth *en bas*, with the palms turned inwards towards each other, the thumb and first finger touching each other, and the hands about six inches apart. Then during the progress of the sequence, the hands rise upwards to the level of the waist, then open outwards, the palms opening out and turning downwards as the arms open; they then close again to the position they were in at first, ready for the next movement upwards. During the whole of this movement the hands describe a sort of figure-of-eight as they turn out after rising, and turn down as they are lowered. The wrists must be supple, and the movement must be timed to take up exactly the same time as the *minuet* step. This movement is done by the gentleman alone, the lady confining herself to holding her dress on either side with her thumb and forefinger, and moving her shoulders wherever epaulement is necessary or appropriate.

Arm Movements for the Presenting of Arms

At the presenting of arms, the movement is different from the above. Whichever hand is presented, the free hand must rise to the second position, with the elbow a little curved and the palm turned forwards. This applies to the lady as well as to the gentleman, but the gentleman may at the same time doff his hat, and hold it out

HISTORICAL DANCES FOR THE THEATRE

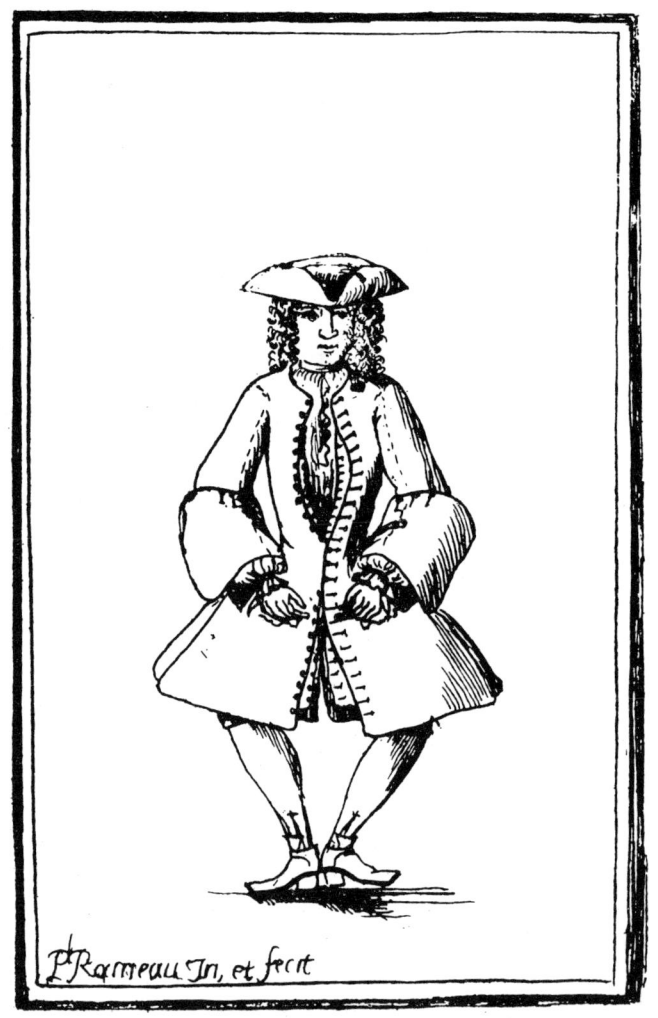

Troisieme tems des bras du Menuet

THE MINUET AND ORNAMENTAL STEPS—LATER PERIOD

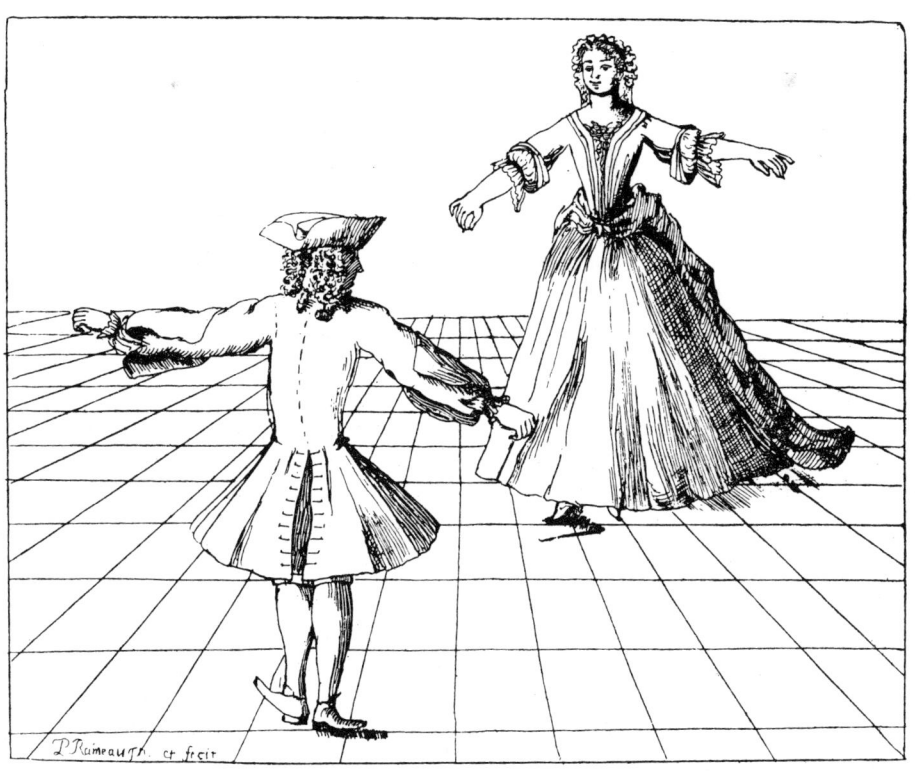

until the figure is complete. Tomlinson thinks this a matter of personal taste, but he is of the opinion that it is more polite and respectful to the lady to remove it. In any case, it must be removed when making the bows before and after the dance.

Arm Movements for the Ornamental Steps

The arm movements for the ornamental steps are more complex, and need some care in studying them before they can be made instinctively with the steps to which they fit. They are based on the principle of 'opposition'. That is to say, the arms move in opposition to the legs, just as they do in walking and running movements. The arms must be held out in a position midway between the first and the second position, with the thumbs and first fingers touching; and whichever foot moves forward, so must the opposite arm move forward and upward in a gentle curve, with an upward turn of the wrist to complete the movement, and a downward turn of the other wrist. The head must turn a little towards the raised arm. When a sequence of several rapid movements is performed, the arms must not move for each little step, as this would look undignified and fussy, beside being very awkward to accomplish; they must move for the most important step in the sequence, and remain still for the others. For instance, in performing the *flying bourrée*, it is on the first step with the bend and rise that the opposition movement is made, and afterwards maintained for the other two steps. In the *balancé* and the *slip* and *half coupée*, the arms move in opposition to the first step sideways, and after that do not move until the sequence is completed. With the *marchés*, the arms move in opposition to each step. The *contretemps* and the *double bourrée* alone are exceptions to this rule, and must therefore be explained separately.

In the *contretemps* both wrists must turn over and downwards with the first small hop, and return to position in the ensuing step; then, with the last bound, the arms simultaneously bend in and downwards as the wrists did previously, but in a larger movement, to correspond with the larger movement of the legs. In the *double bourrée*, the wrists turn in and downwards simultaneously on the first step to the side, and on the last step, when the right foot is drawn up to the third position back, the right wrist turns upwards again to form a slight opposition.

These movements of the arms and wrists should be practised until they are soft and flowing, and they should also be practised with *minuet* steps between, so that the arm movements that belong to the ornamental steps can be made to flow easily and naturally into those of the *minuet*.

THE MINUET AND ORNAMENTAL STEPS—LATER PERIOD

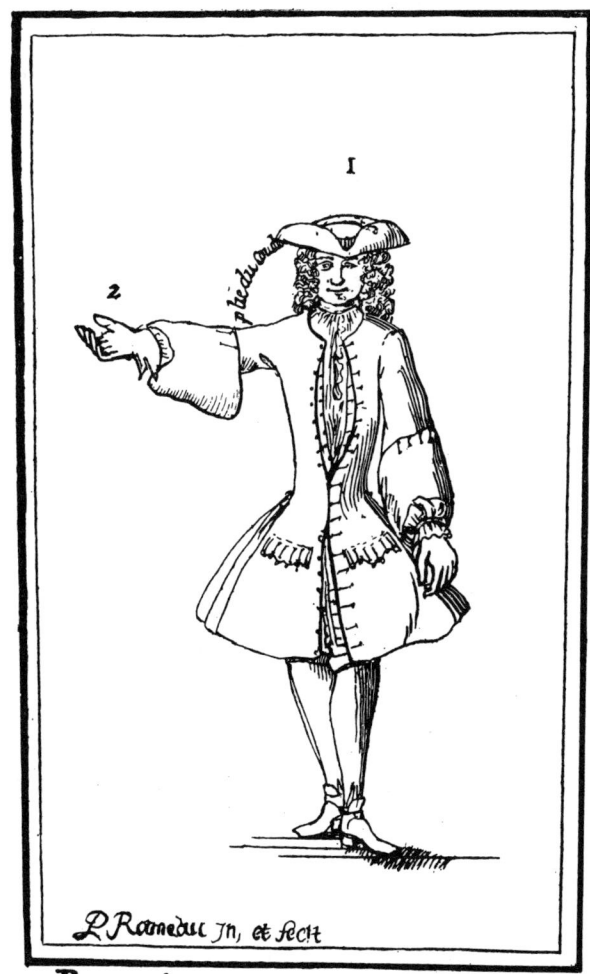

Premiere tems pour oster le Chapeau

OBSERVATIONS ON STYLE

IT IS IMPOSSIBLE to convey in writing the exact style in which a dance should be performed, especially one so full of subtle nuances of movement and timing as the Minuet, and dancers must use their imagination in turning these dry instructions into terms of movement and music. Nevertheless, a few words of advice may help to make the foregoing descriptions a little clearer, and give a general view of the whole dance as it should be when performed, complete with all its steps, airs and grace.

First of all, it is important for the legs to be well 'turned out'; this does not mean that it is necessary to be as much turned out as the trained ballet dancer, with the feet in a straight line, but the more turned out the legs and feet are, the easier the steps will be to perform, and the better the balance and carriage. In the seventeenth century, professional dancers began to realise the advantages of being turned out, and that Mlle. Camargo was more turned out than her teacher, is significant of an increase in technical accomplishment.

The instep should be strong and supple, to enable the dancer to execute the innumerable bends and rises smoothly, and without effort. The knees must bend only in the larger movements, but the instep flexes with every step. For example, the first bend and rise of the French *minuet* step is done with the instep only, and the succeeding bends and rises are done with the knees as well as the insteps. When a step is described as being done on the toes, this should be taken as meaning on half point. In executing such steps as the *flying bourrée*, the last two steps should be done on the toes without lowering the heels, and the steps should be small and neat. Rameau writes, 'The more steps you perform *sur le demi-point*, the lighter you will appear to be'.

The body should be held erect but easy, and the steps made smoothly and evenly without sudden jolts on the bounds, or on the bends and rises; and, when one foot is crossed before the other in the execution of a step sideways, the opposite shoulder should be turned forward as the step is made. The lady, being occupied in holding her dress, and therefore unable to use her hands while dancing, should learn to move her shoulders gracefully in *epaulement*.

The gaze should be directed at the partner wherever possible, but as in certain figures the dancers are momentarily back to back, such as the Z figures, where they pass one another, the head should be turned towards that side on which they have passed each other, and then turned to face again as soon as it is possible to do so with grace and dignity. In the ornamental steps, the head is turned

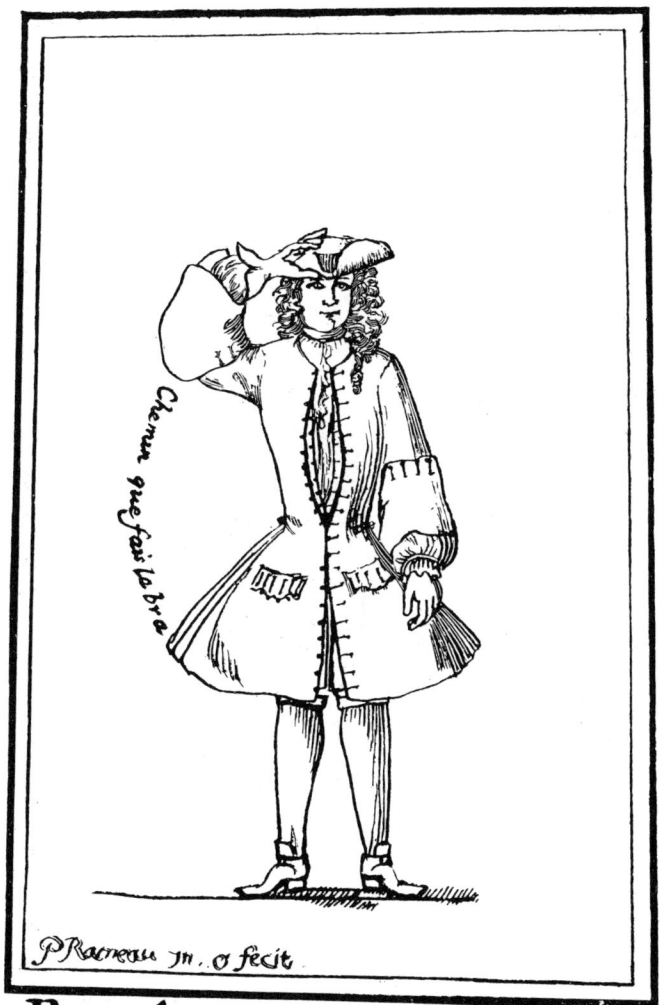

Deuxieme attitude de
l'exercisse du Chapeau

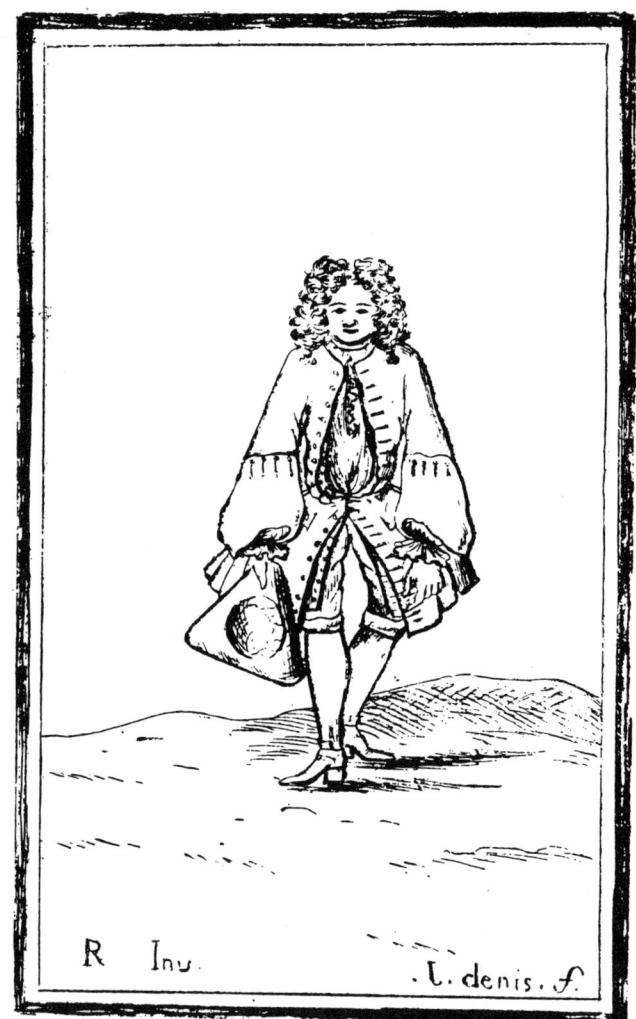

Deuxieme Figure Inclinée veüe de face

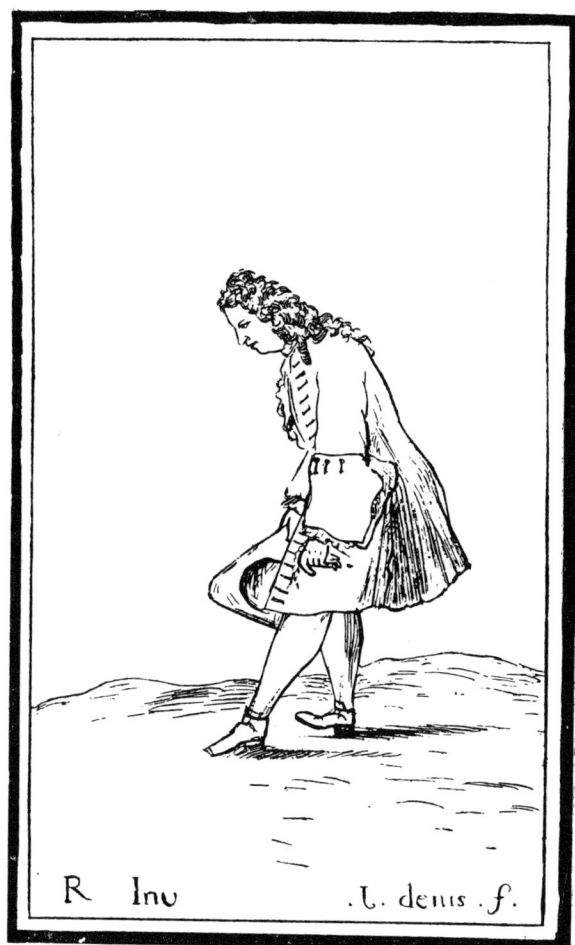

Deuxieme Figure Inclinée et veüe de profil

towards the hand that is in opposition, and this should be cultivated carefully, as it prevents monotony, and gives added variety to the dance.

The figures should be symmetrical and well balanced, and the gentleman should always match his steps to the lady's, especially in the *contretemps* and the *passepied* steps, where bounds occur. The lady may not bound high, even if she can, as it is not in keeping with the style, and so the gentleman must make his bounds as small and neat as hers.

It is impossible to pretend that the Minuet is an easy dance for anyone but an accomplished dancer to perform properly, and the amateur will be well advised to learn first to do it without any of the ornamental steps. Tomlinson says that he has seen unskilled dancers go the whole course of the dance, executing their steps across the bars, through making a false start; and he also says that if a dancer is not sufficiently experienced to be able to maintain the rhythm of the dance, and at the same time introduce ornamental steps, he should content himself with dancing it with the *minuet* step exclusively.

THE DOUBLE HONOURS

BEFORE and after the dance the lady and gentleman are expected to make two bows, one to the spectators or the Presence, and one to each other. The bows are performed in this manner: the gentleman takes the lady's left hand in his right, and leads her to the bottom of the room. They turn to face the Presence, and the gentleman, removing his hat with his left hand, they execute the following movements simultaneously. Place the inside foot in the fourth position in front *pointe tendue*, slide it to the second position on the flat of the foot so that the weight is equally distributed, and bow to the Presence. The lady does this by bending both knees in a *plié*, and the gentleman does it by bending forward from the waist. They then *dégagé* the outside foot, slide it to the third position behind, step forward, and a little away from one another with the inside foot, and bring the outside foot round in a semi-circle to the second position, facing each other. The lady then closes the inside foot to the first position, and the gentleman closes the inside foot to the third position behind, after which they bow as before. The gentleman then replaces his hat and they are ready to begin the dances. The same bows are done at the end of the dance, with or without music. It is better to do them without music in both cases, or in the case of the first bows, to play the first strain an extra time, so that the first *minuet* step may afterwards be made with the commencement of the tune. Tomlinson provides special introductory music for the bows in his Minuets, but this is exceptional.

A SUMMARY OF THE FEUILLET DANCE NOTATION IN RELATION TO THE MINUET

AS THE EXAMPLE of the Minuet is written in notation, it is necessary to understand the few signs that are used in writing it out. The table which is given below shows the signs used to indicate the track of the dance, bends, rises, bounds, slides, turns, etc. With the assistance of these, the various ornamental steps and the dance itself, will be understood more clearly. Some of the ornamental steps will be found more difficult to understand than others, notably the early *contretemps* and the late *fleuret*, but a careful study of the signs will make them intelligible, and the following hints will be found useful.

Foot in Air Sign

It will be seen that the sign for lifting, or keeping the foot in the air, is marked in two different places. When the sign is marked at the end of the step, it indicates that the foot must be raised and held up, and when the sign is marked in the middle of the step, the foot must be raised and afterwards put down. Both these movements are demonstrated in the *contretemps*.

Turning Signs

The signs for turning on a step should be observed carefully, as these affect the direction of the ensuing steps. The direction of a turn is easily remembered if it is kept in mind that it is always made in the opposite direction from the side on which its beginning is marked. Notice carefully when a step crosses the track, as this may indicate that a turn is there, or that the foot which is moving goes behind or in front of the other foot.

Bends, Bounds and Hops

Where a bend is marked before a bound, it is not necessary to make a special movement of this: It is obviously impossible to make any sort of jumping movement without bending the knees a little, and this sign is marked whenever a bound or a hop occurs. On the last position marked in the *Pas de Mons. Marcel*, no bend is marked, and this is correct, as the movement is more a drop on to the foot than a bound. In any case, a deep bend before a small bound can only have the effect of making the whole movement heavy. Certain alterations have been made in writing out some of the steps in notation to make them more intelligible to the uninitiated, but without altering the steps themselves in any way.

Rests

In the *balancé* and the *slip* and *half coupée* there are rest signs; these are used as in music, and no movement is to be made where they are marked. Their values are noted under the signs in the table.

The Fifth Position

Professional dancers studying these directions and diagrams, may notice that the fifth position is never mentioned, for although it was accounted for among the positions of the feet when these were first formulated, it was rarely used, and the third position took its place. The professional dancers of the seventeenth and eighteenth century were not as much turned out as they are to-day, and the third position was more natural for them than the fifth. In spite of this, it must not be supposed that they were unable to perform difficult and brilliant technical feats.

Entrechats and *pirouettes* were known to them, and, if one may trust contemporary writers, executed brilliantly by the famous dancers of the Paris Opera. For the benefit of those people who imagine that these things were only being discovered in our own times, it may be of interest to know that not only were these same steps known to sixteenth century dancers, but such brilliant technical feats as *deux tours en l'air*, were also known to them. This last movement was not used by the dancers of the seventeenth century, and it only appears again in classical ballet later in the eighteenth century.

INDEX TO PLATES FOLLOWING

PLATE I	A Table of Signs	53
PLATE II	The Minuet Step—Early Period	54
PLATE III	Ornamental Steps—Early Period	55
PLATE IV	The Minuet Step—Later Period	56
PLATE V	Ornamental Steps—Later Period	57

The Minuet:

PLATE VI	Figure 1—Introduction	58
PLATE VII	Figure 2—The S Reversed	59
PLATE VIII	Figure 3—The Presenting of the Right Hand	60
PLATE IX	Figure 4—The Presenting of the Left Hand	61
PLATE X	Figure 5—The S Reversed	62
PLATE XI	Figure 6—The Presenting of both Hands	63

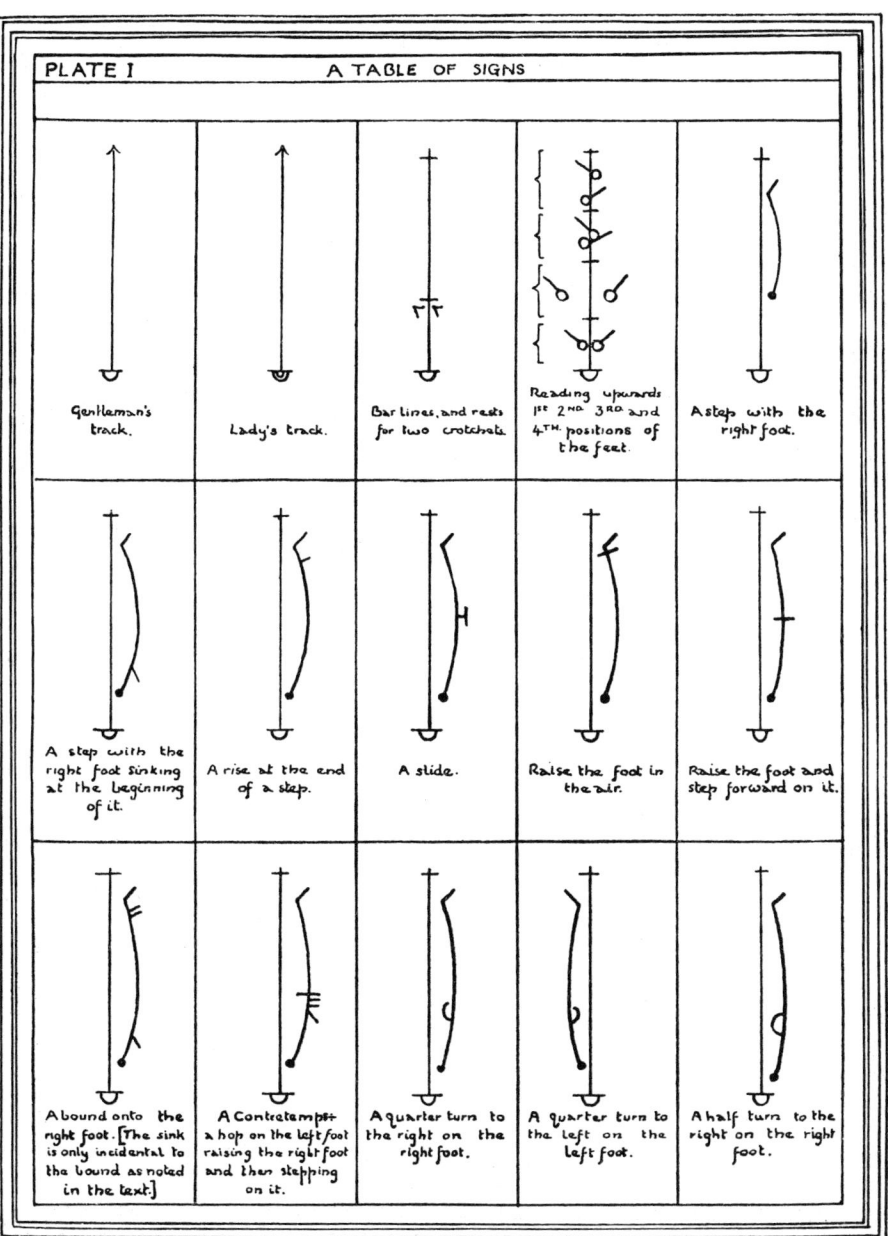

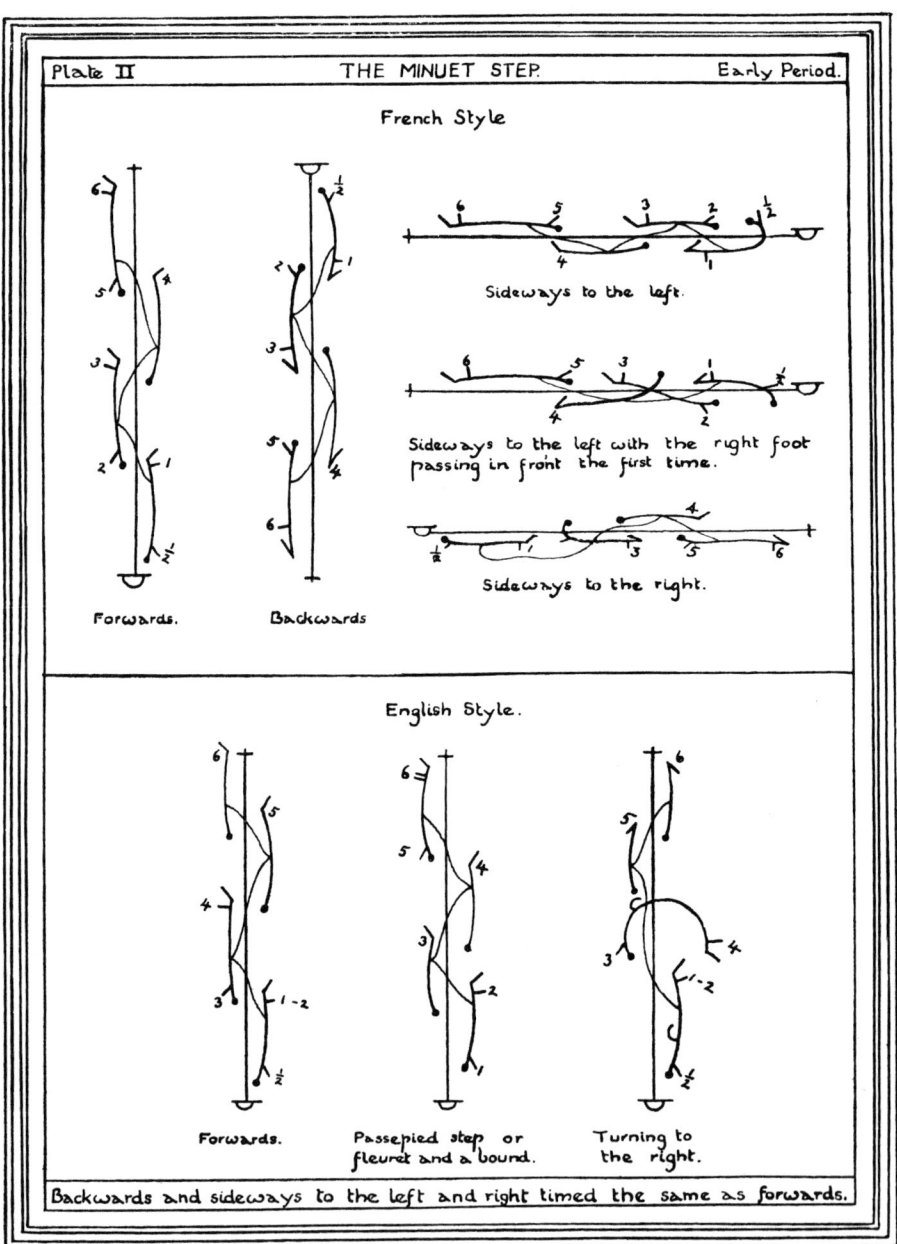

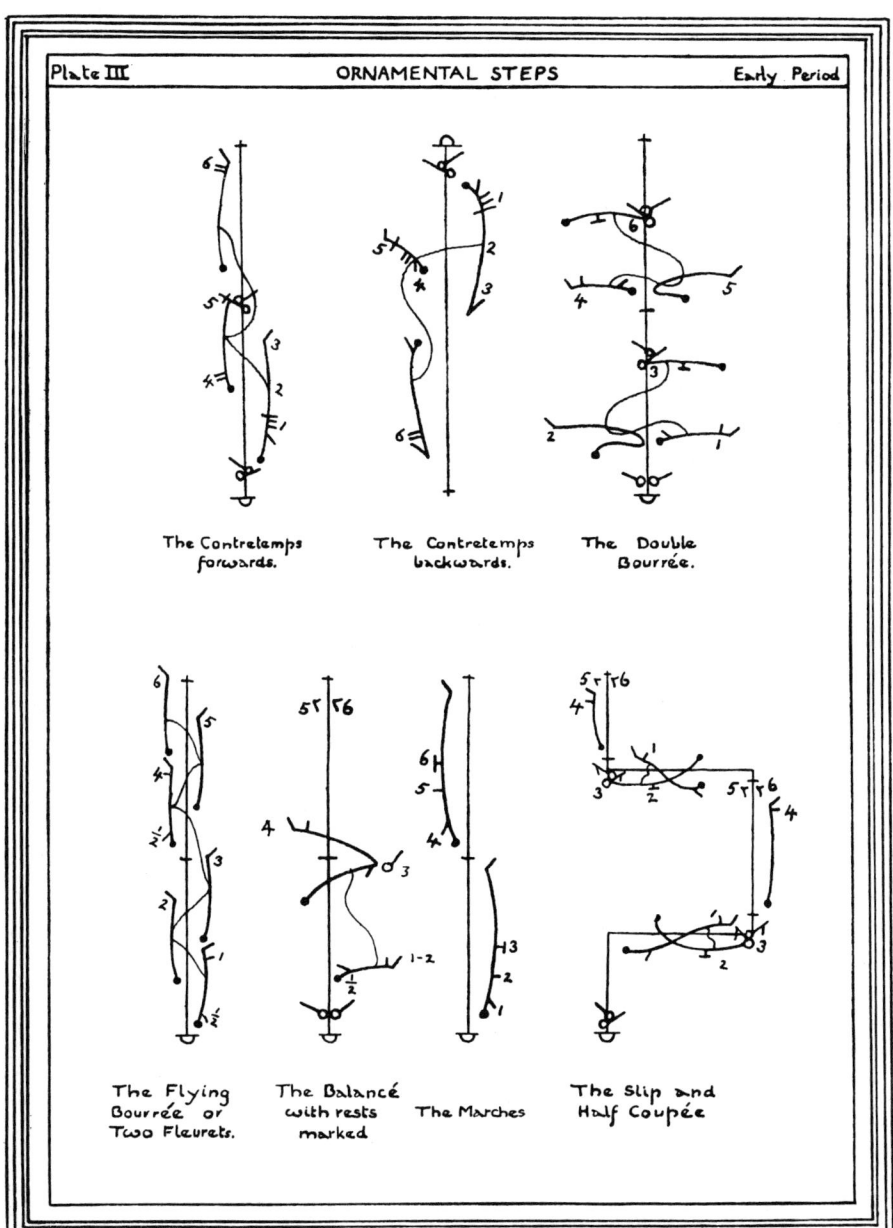

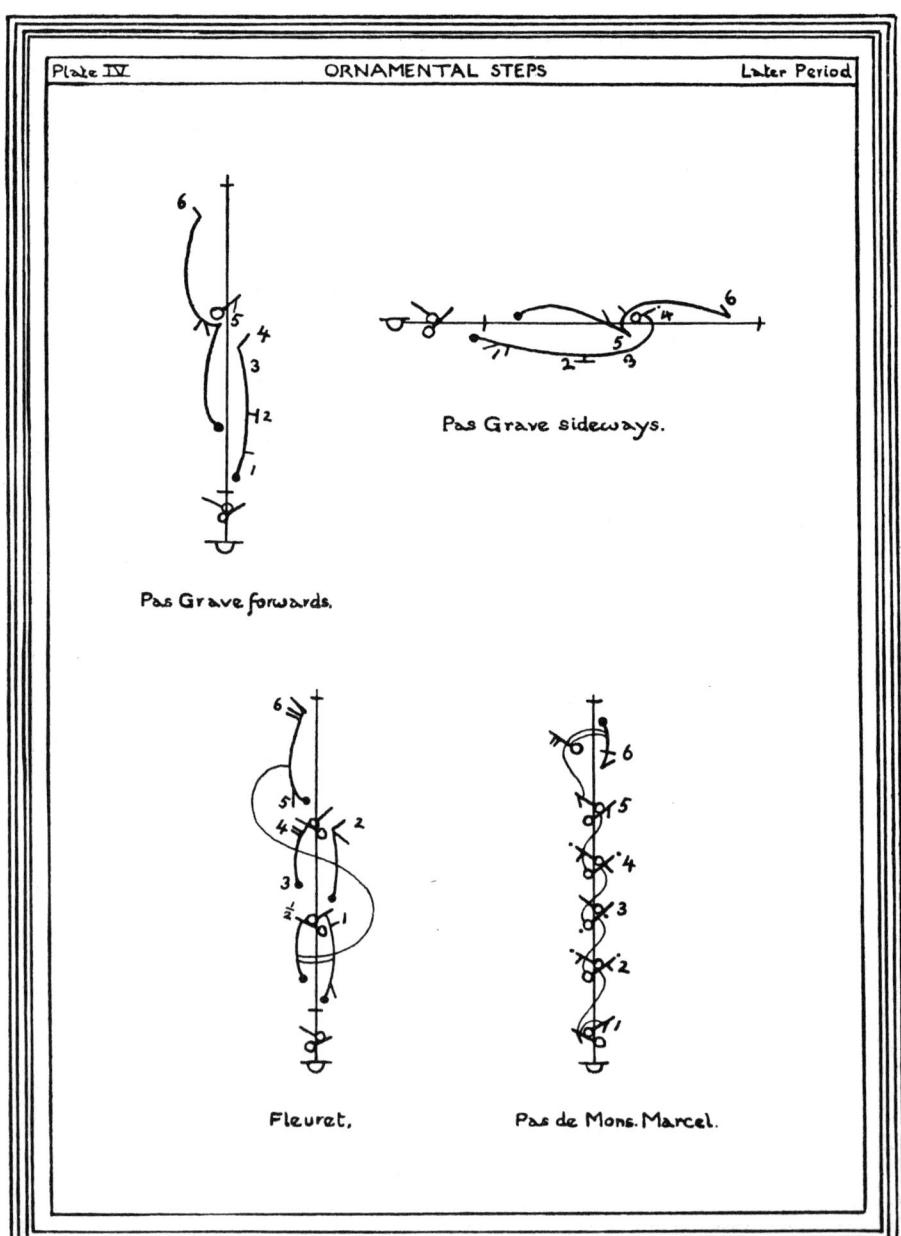

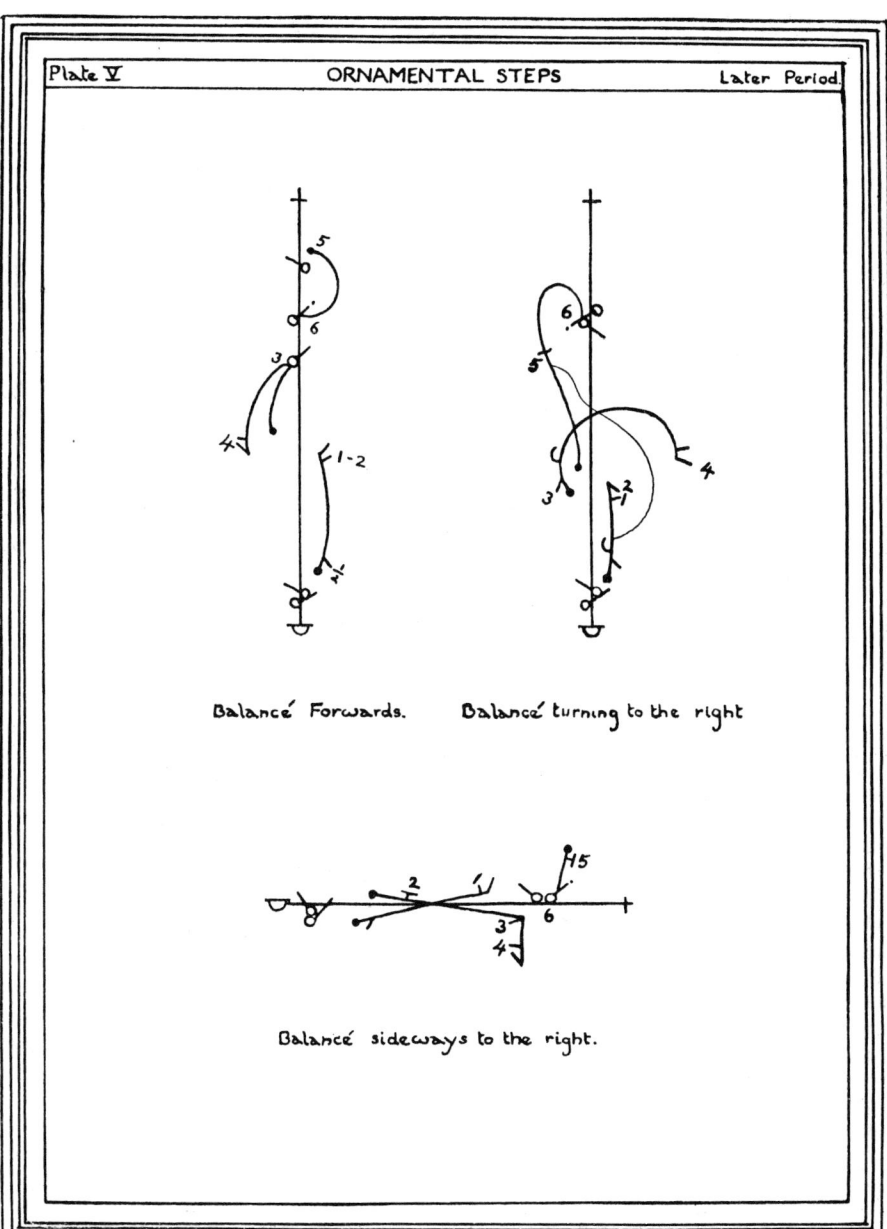

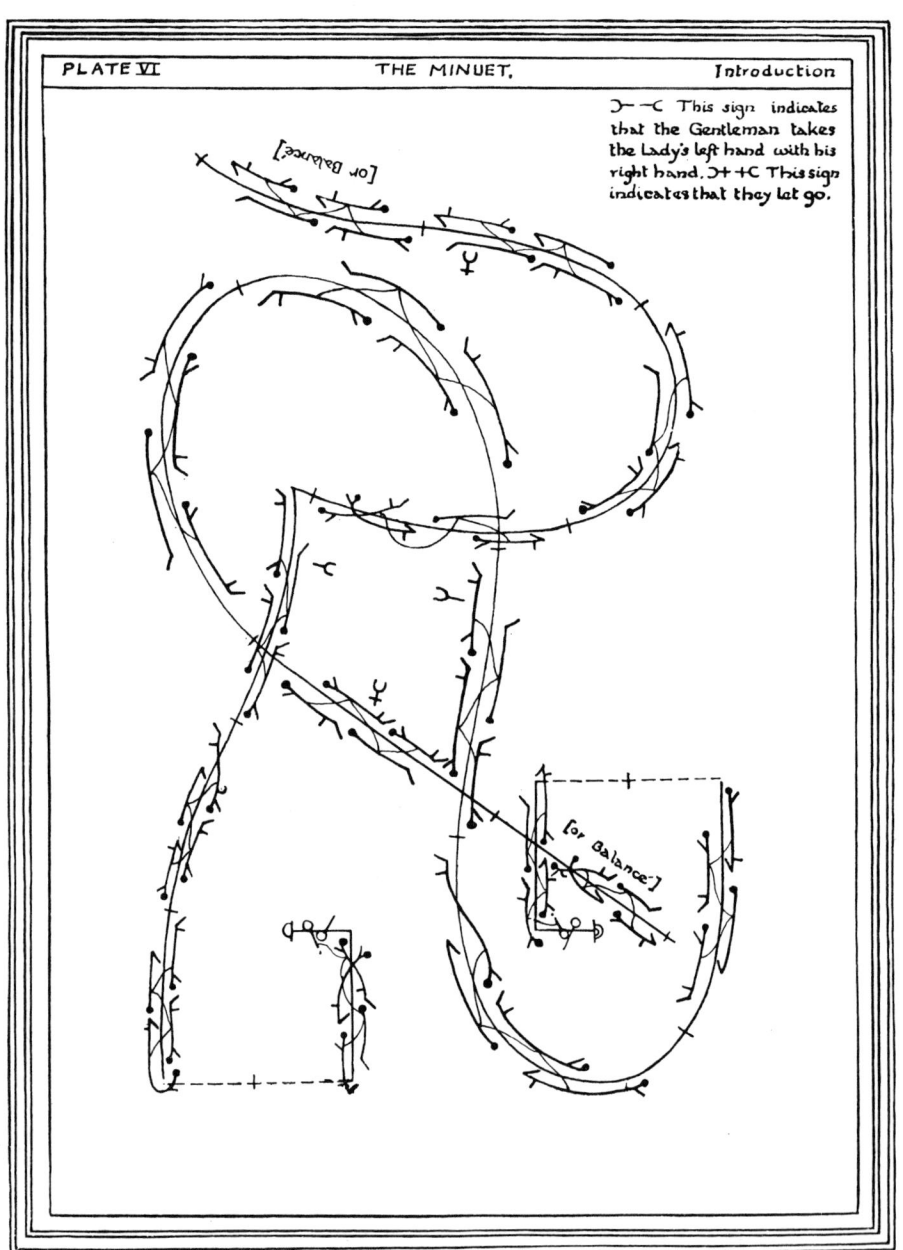

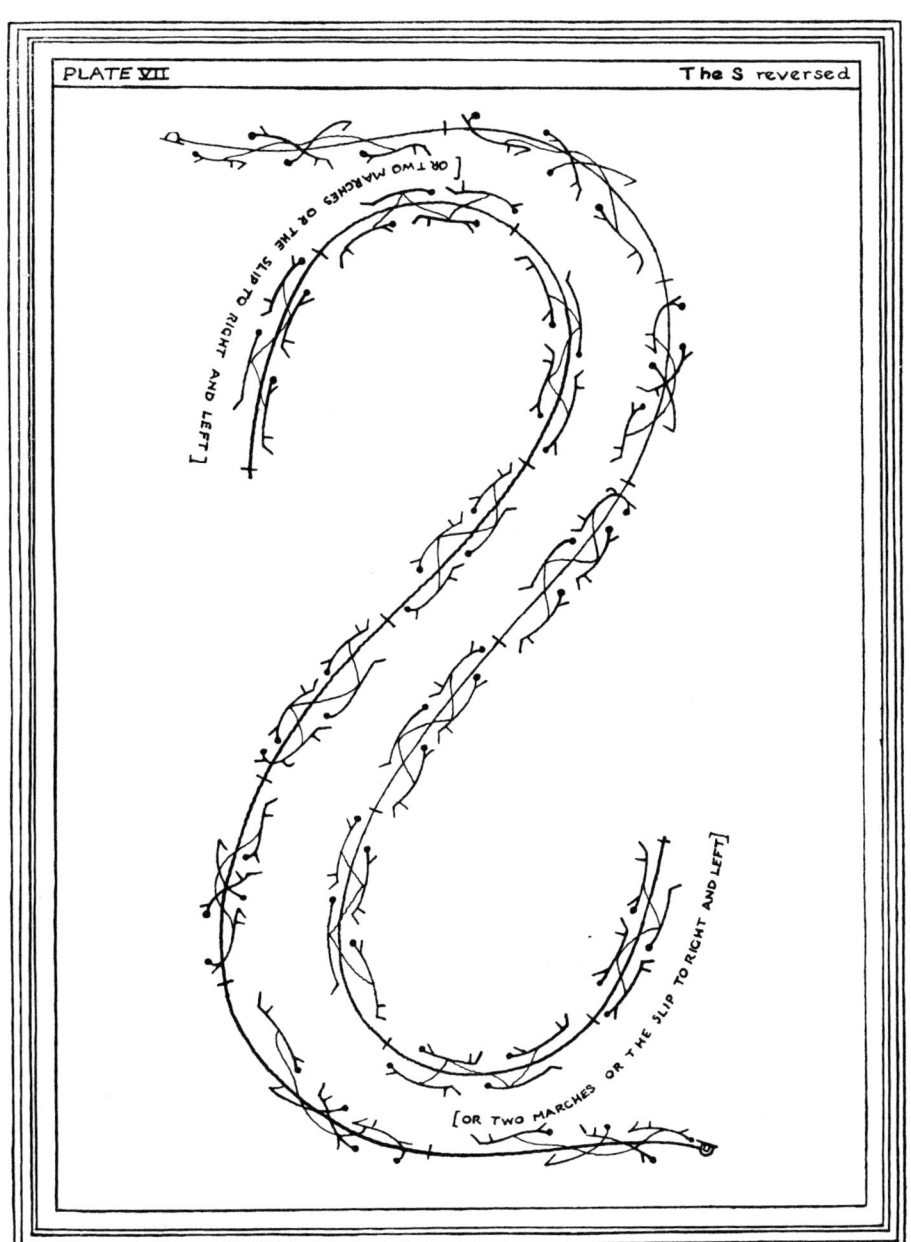

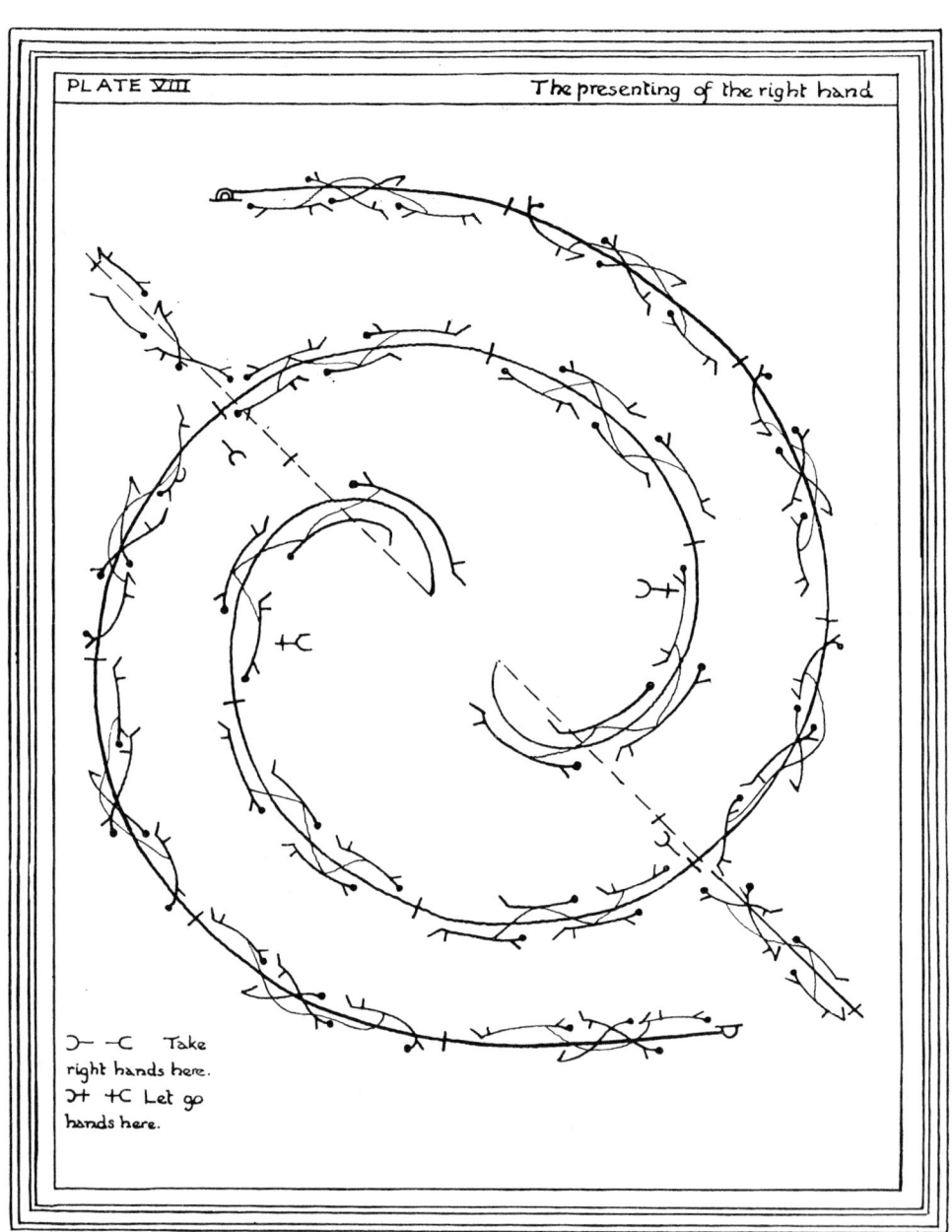

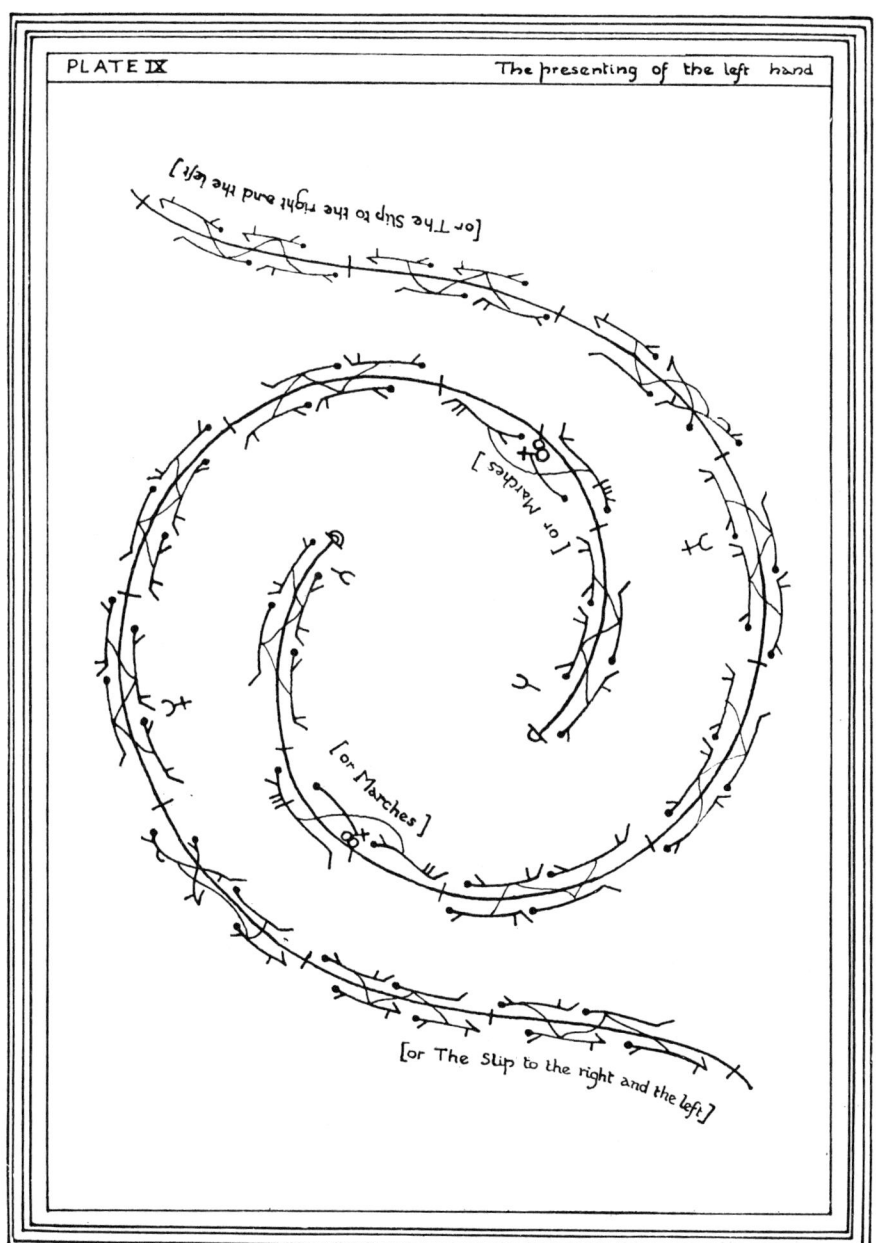

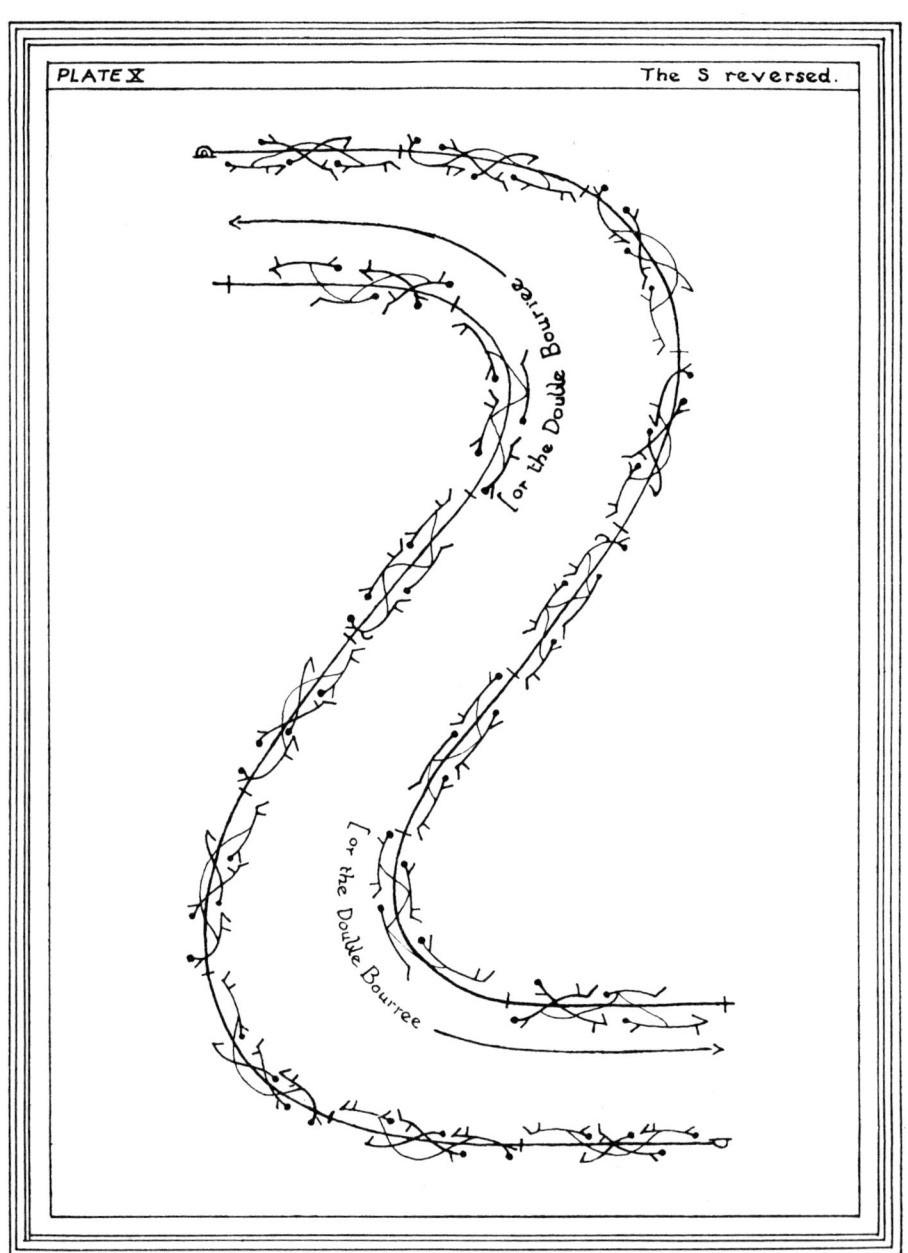

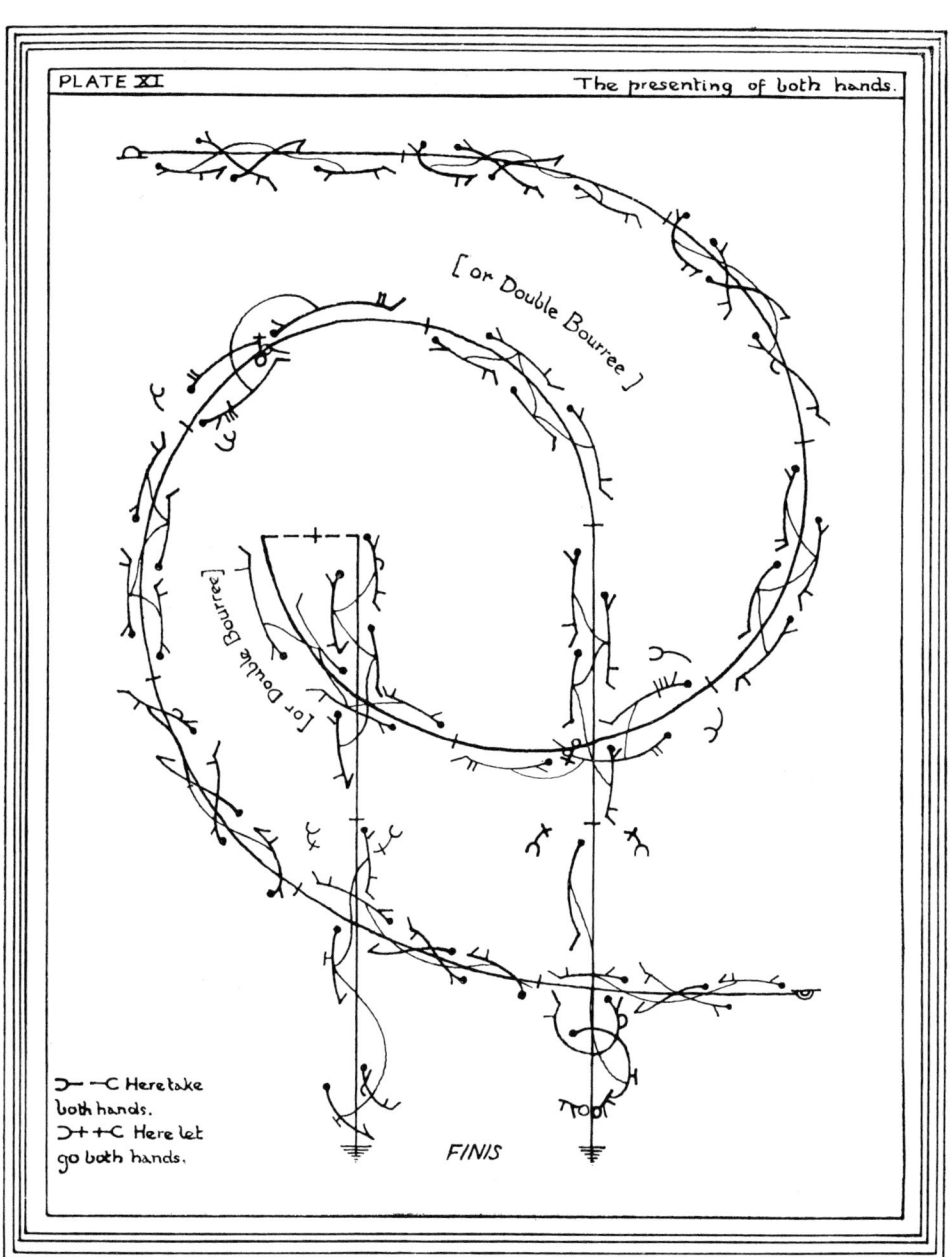

MUSIC

Pavana Bray

William Byrd

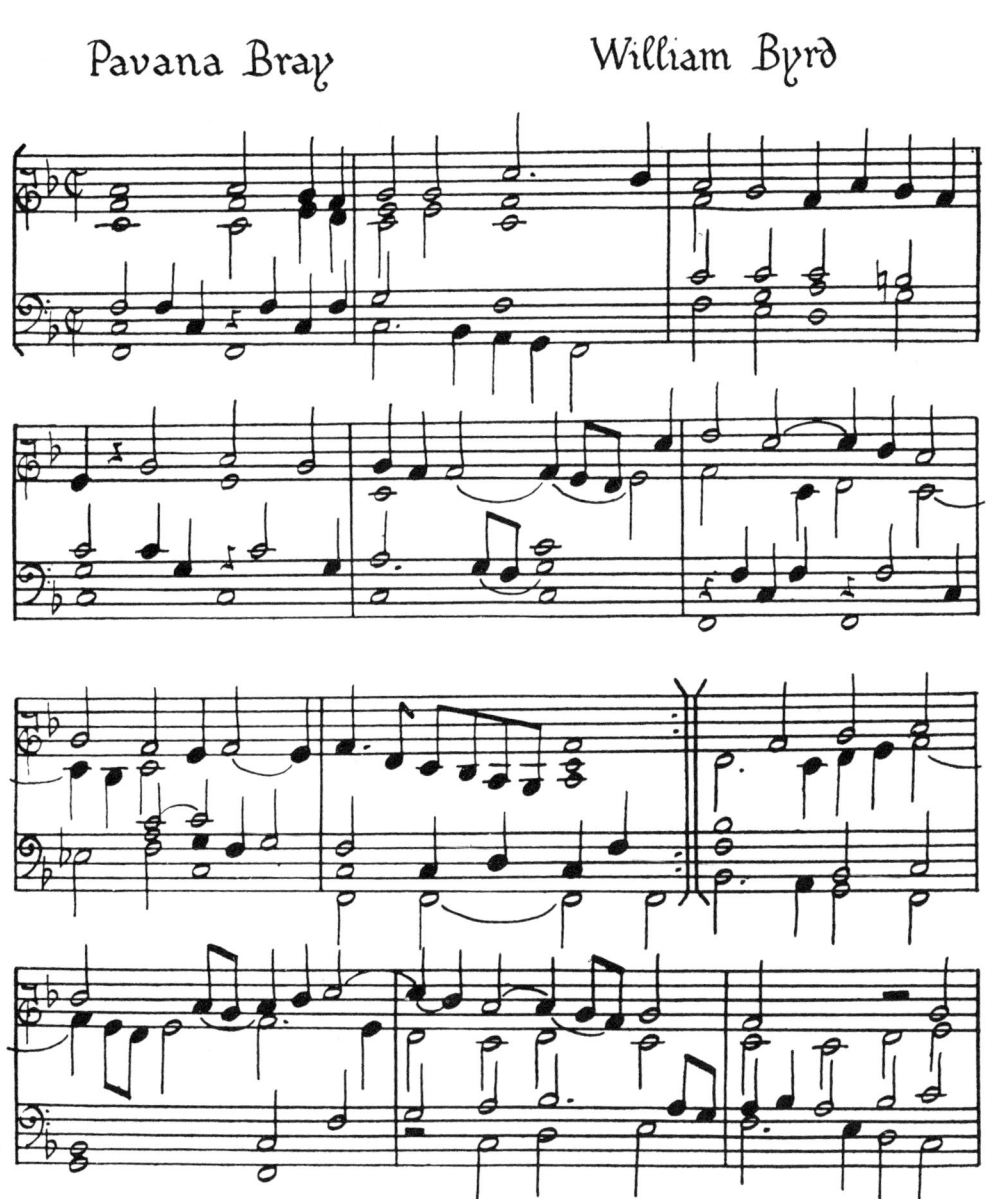

Pavana Bray (cont) — William Byrd

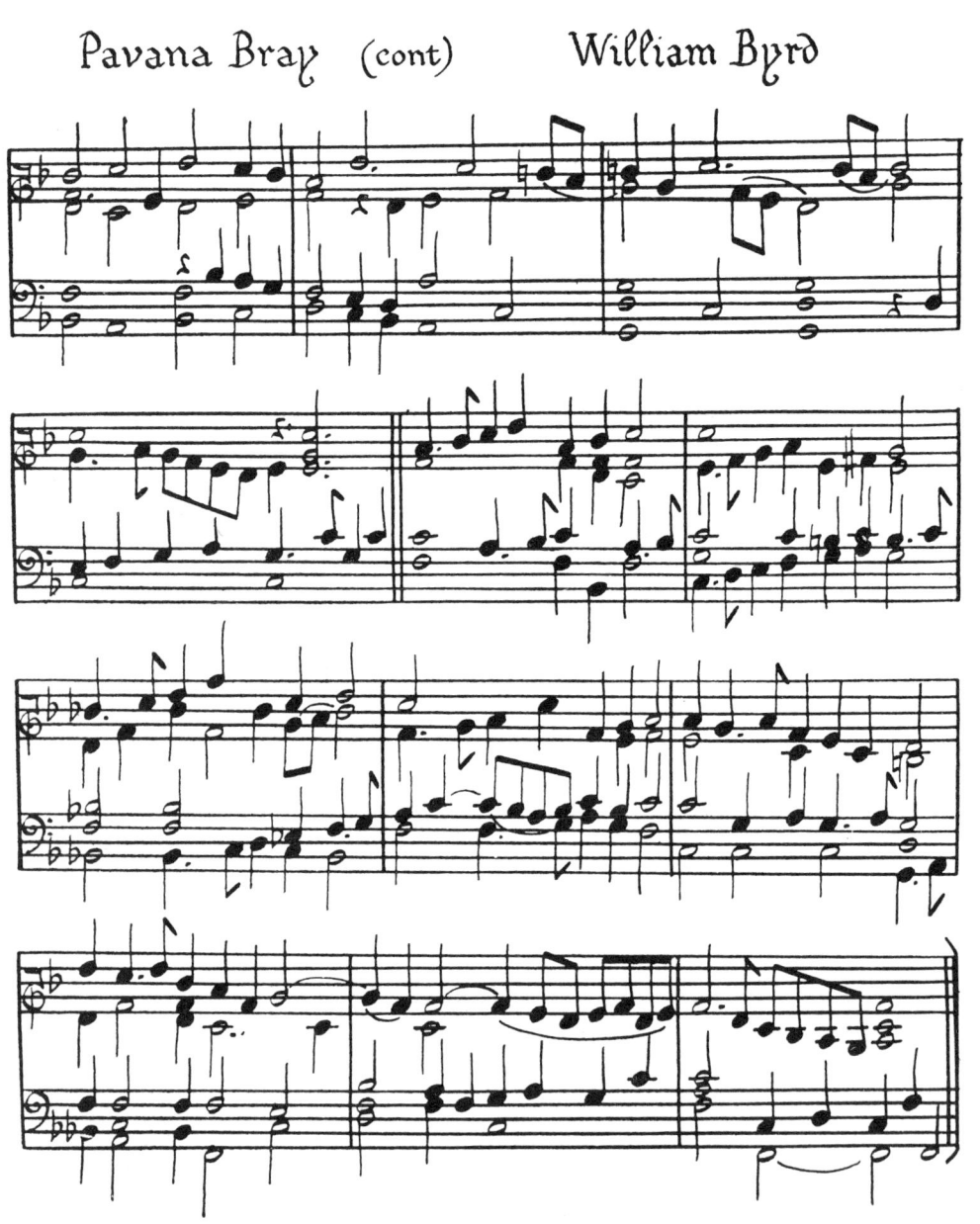

Pavan
Luys Milan 1535

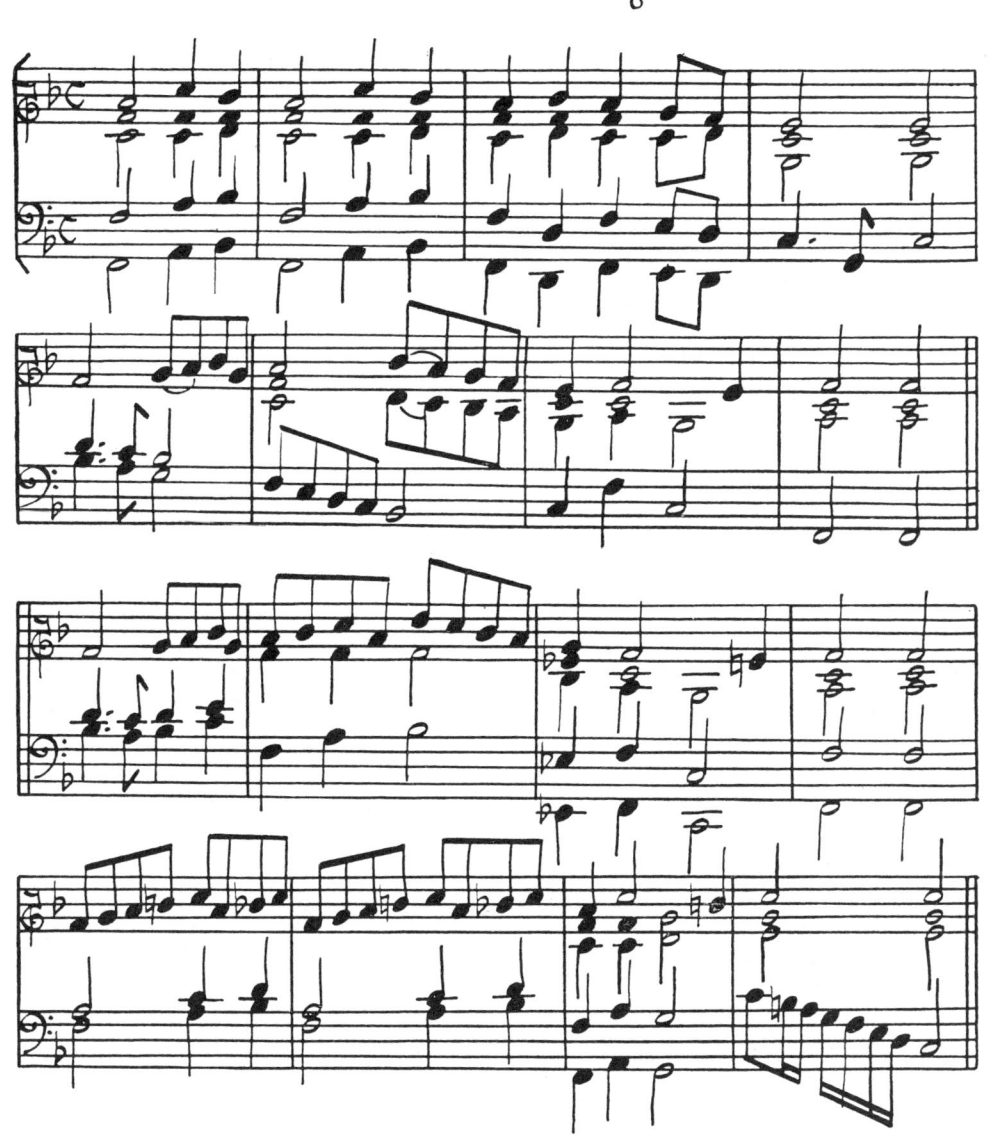

Pavan (cont) — Luys Milan 1535

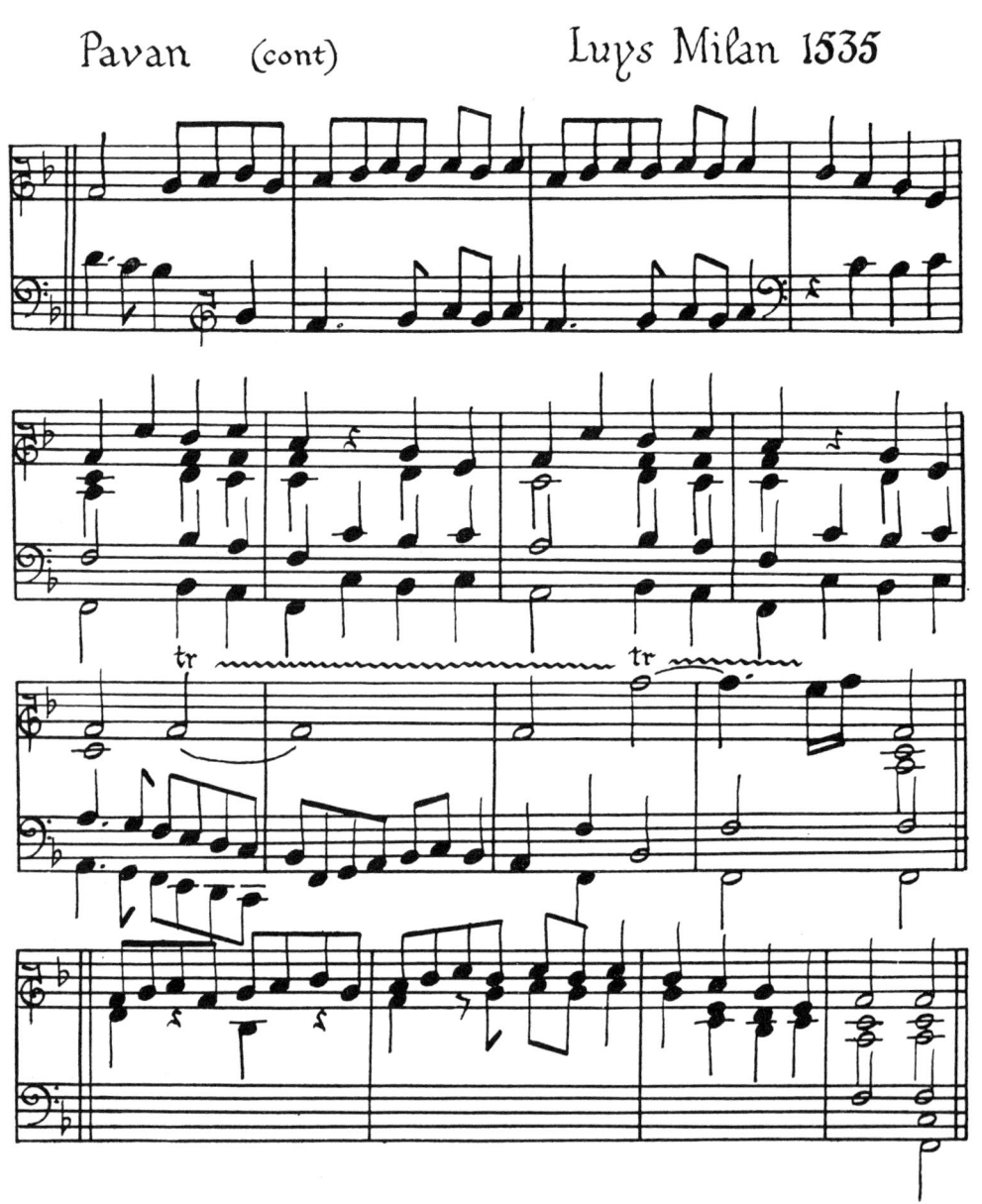

Pavan (cont) — Luys Milan 1535

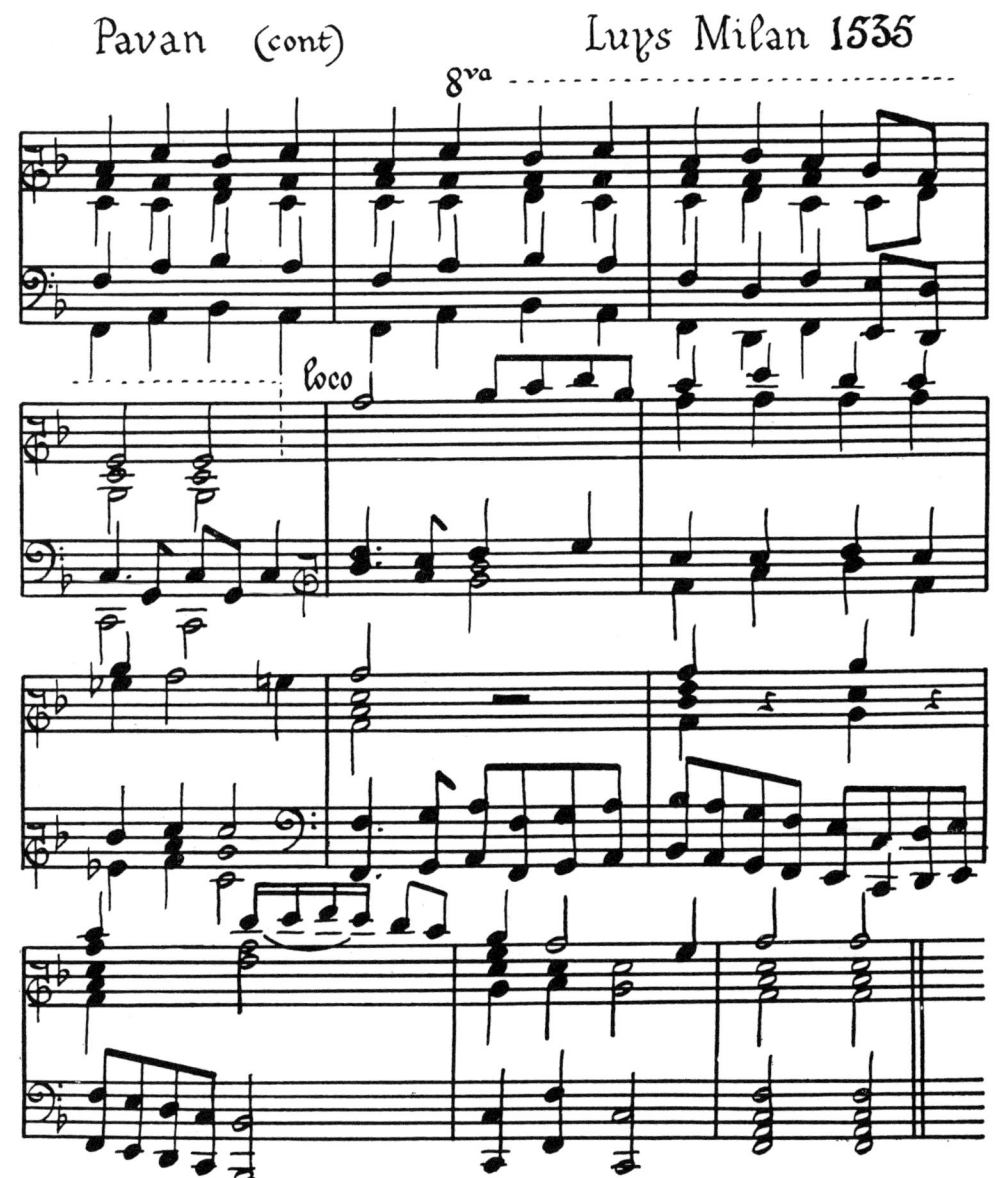

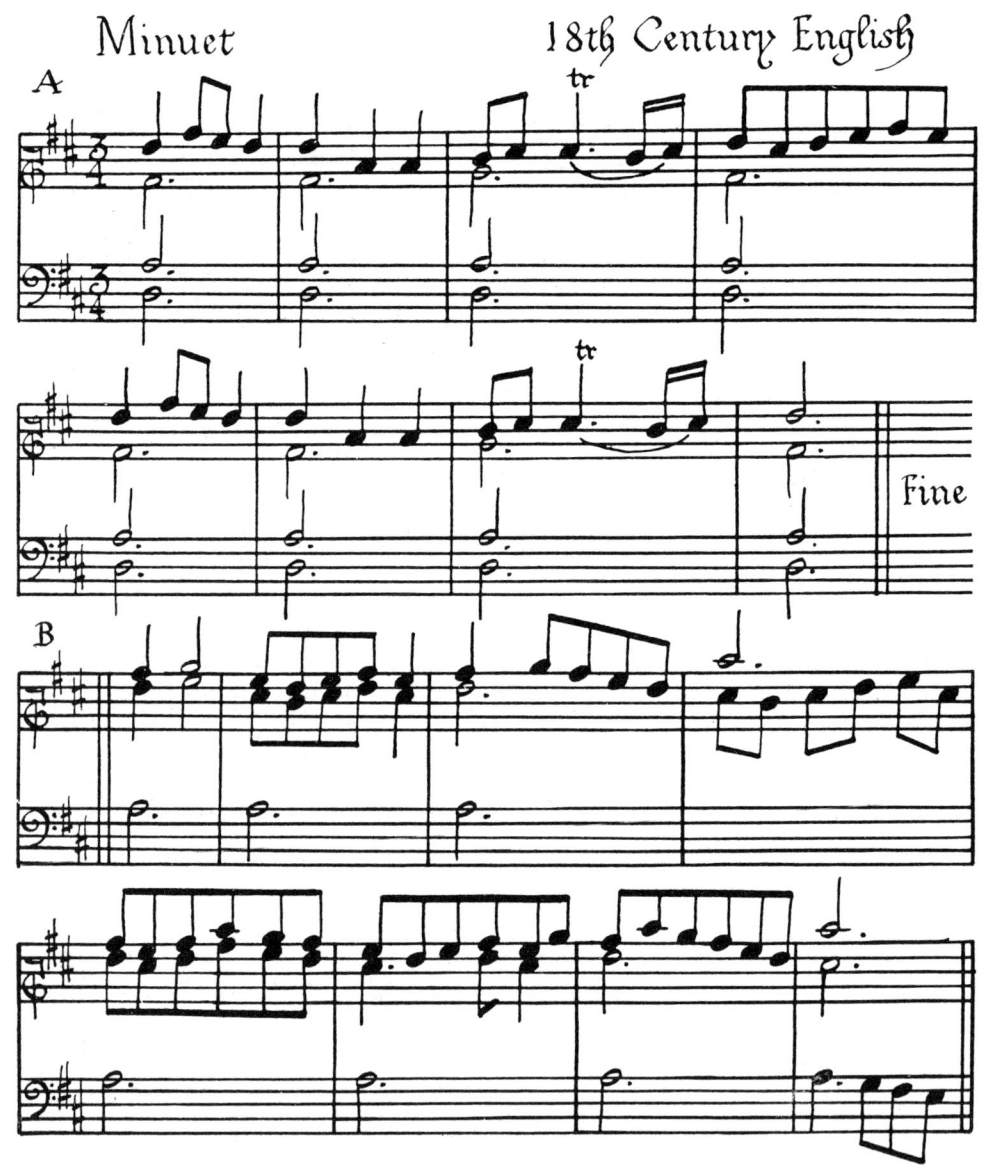

Minuet (cont) — 18th Century English

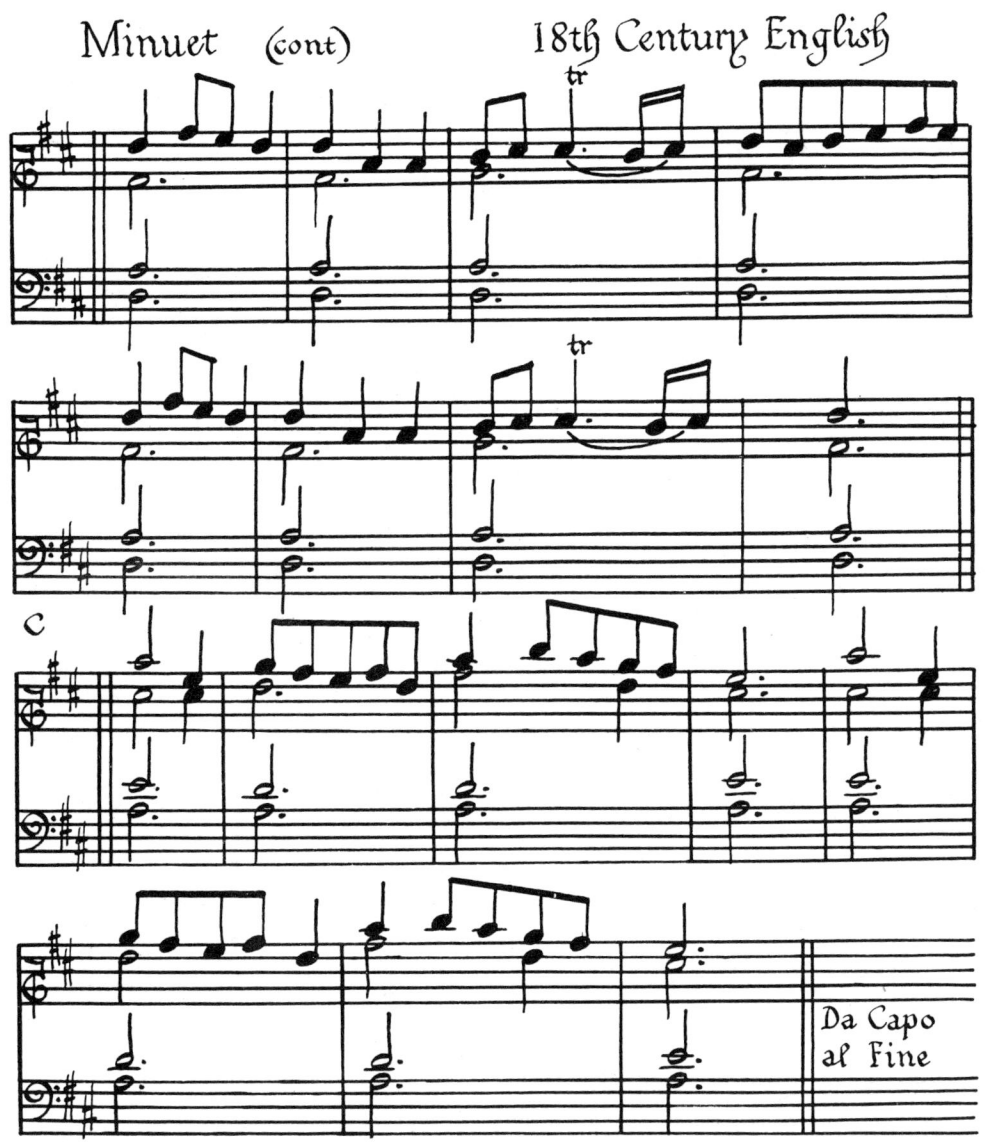

Deux Passepieds
Jean Joseph Mouret 1730

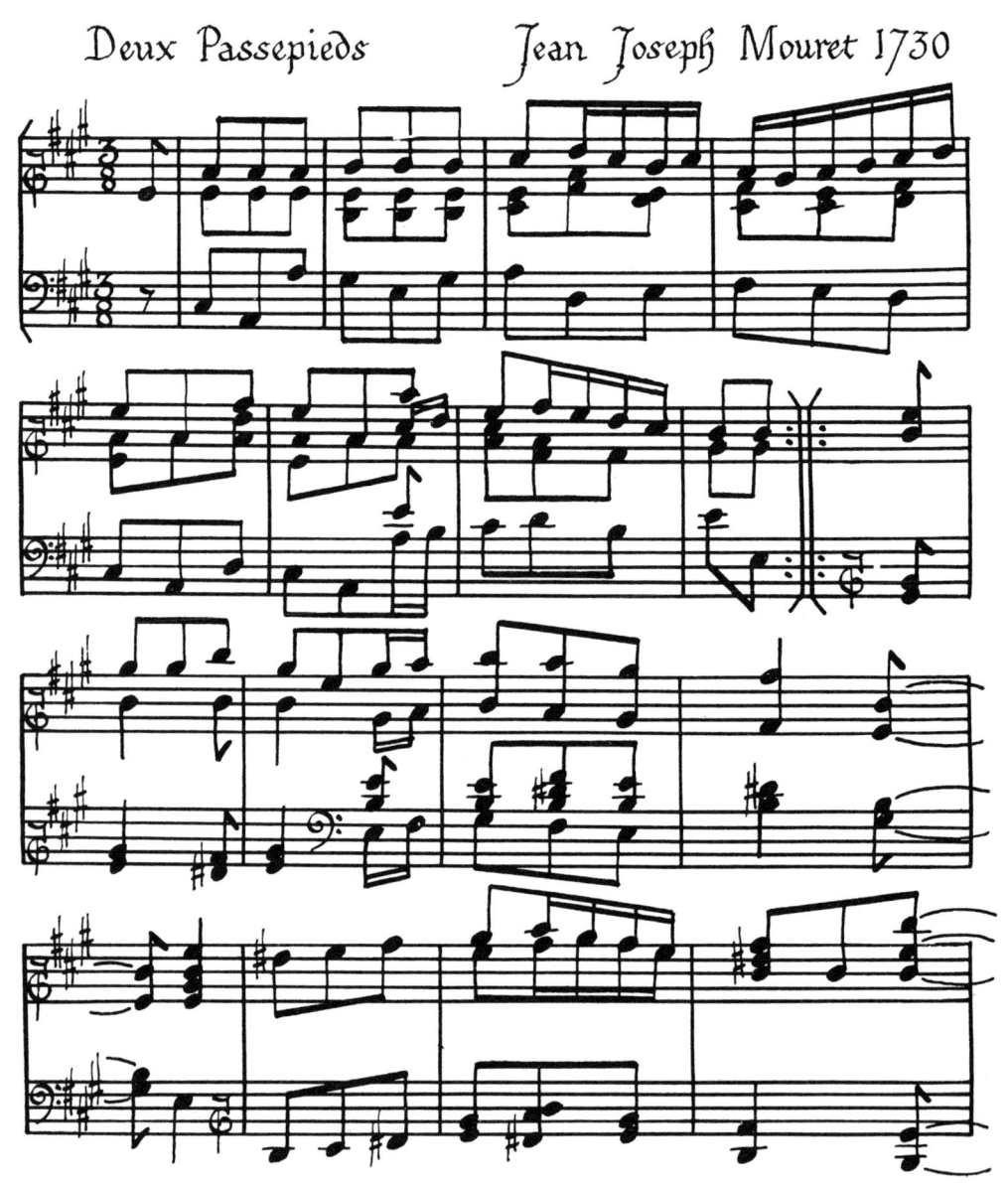

Deux Passepieds (cont) — Jean Joseph Mouret 1730

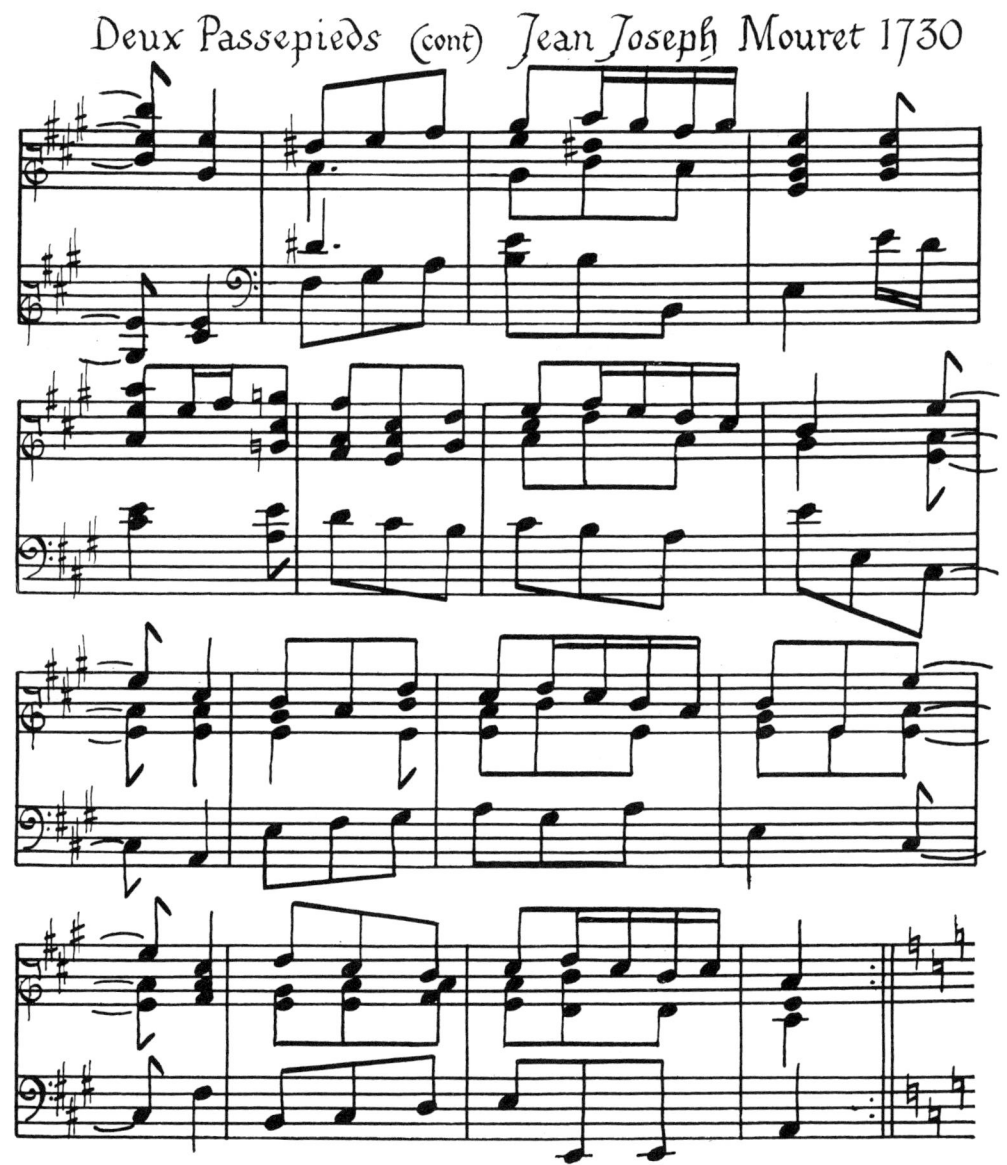

Deux Passepieds (cont) Jean Joseph Mouret 1730

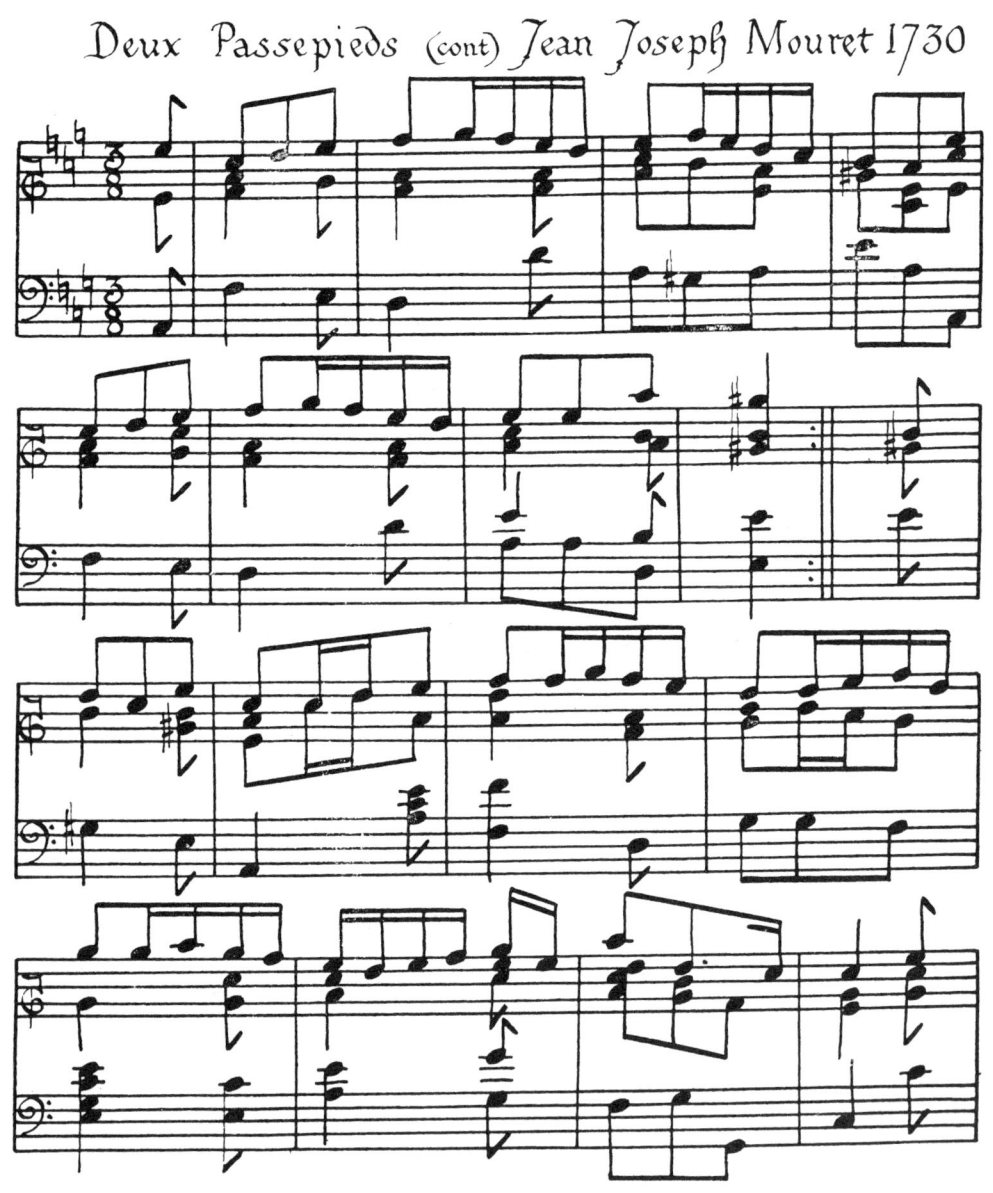

Deux Passepieds (cont) Jean Joseph Mouret 1730

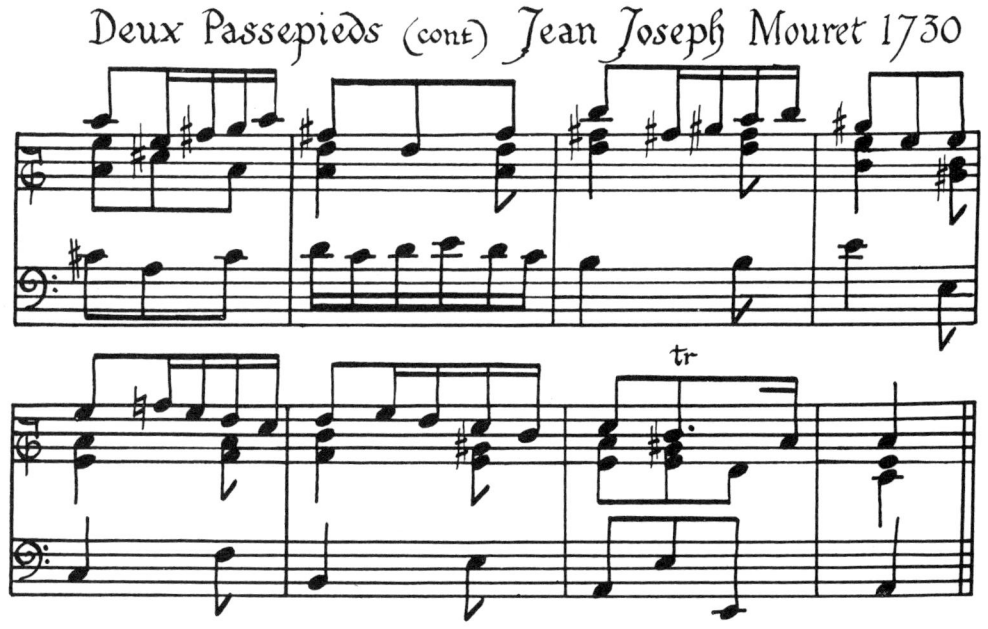

BIBLIOGRAPHY

A SHORT LIST of the principal authorities consulted for the purposes of this book. The reference numbers are from the British Museum catalogue unless otherwise stated. The books are arranged in chronological order except for translations which follow the original.

Trattato Dell'arte Del Ballo. Guglielmo Ebreo da Pesaro. Circa 1460. Bibliothèque Nationale, Paris.
L'art et l'instruction de Bien Dancer. Published by Michel Toulouze. Paris, circa 1488. Library of the Royal College of Physicians. Reprinted in facsimile 1936. Ref. 07908, f. 42.
The Manner To Daunce Bace Daunces. Published by Robert Coplande. London 1521. Bodleian Library.
Le Manuscrit Dit Des Basses Danses de la Bibliothèque De Bourgogne. Circa 1523. Bibliothèque Royale, Brussels.
Le Manuscrit Dit Des Basses Danses. Int. et trans. par Ernest Closson. Brussels 1912. Ref. K. 10. a. 28.
. . . Ad Suos Compagnones Studiantes . . . Antonius d'Arena. Lyons? 1529. Ref. 1070. b. 2. (2). Of six editions published this is the first.
Il Ballarino. Fabritio Caroso. Venice 1581. Ref. 558* c. 17.
Orchesographie. Thoinot Arbeau. Langres 1588. Ref. C. 31. b. 3.
Orchesography. Thoinot Arbeau. Translation by Cyril W. Beaumont. London 1925. Ref. C. 100. g. 13.
Nobiltà di Dame. Fabritio Caroso. Venice 1600. Ref. Case 77. d. 12.
Nuove Inventioni Di Balli. Cesare Negri. Milan 1604. Ref. 785. M. 8.
Terpsichore. Michel Praetorius. Wolfenbuttel 1612.
De Harmonie Universelle. Marin Mersenne. Paris 1636. Ref. 558* c. 11.
Choregraphie Ou L'art de D'ecrire la Dance par Caractères, Figures et Signes Demonstratifs. R. A. Feuillet. Paris 1701. Ref. 556. c. 13 (1).
Recueil De Danse. R. A. Feuillet. Paris 1704. Ref. 7895. c. 24.
The Art of Dancing Demonstrated by Characters and Figures. P. Siris. London 1706. Ref. 785. k. 6.
Orchesography, or, The Art of Dancing by Characters and Demonstrative Figures. John Weaver. London 1706. Ref. 558* c. 39.
A Small Treatise of Time and Cadence in Dancing. London 1706. Ref. 785, k. 7. (1).
An Essay for the Further Improvement of Dancing. E. Pemberton. London 1711. Ref. 556, c. 16.
Nouveau Recueil De Danse de Bal et de Celles de Ballet. L. Pécour. Recueilles et Misses Au Jour Par M. Gaudrau. Paris 1712. Bibliothèque Nationale.
Le Maître A Danser. P. Rameau. Paris 1725. Ref. 1042. 1.21.
The Dancing Master. P. Rameau. Translation by Cyril W. Beaumont. London 1931. Ref. C. 100. g. 26.
Abbregé de la Nouvelle Methode dans l'Art D'ecrire ou de Tracer Toutes Sortes de Danses de Ville. P. Rameau. Paris 1725. Ref. C. 31. g. 7.
Trattato Del Ballo Nobile. Giambattista Dufort. Naples 1728. Ref. 1041. c. 9.
The Art of Dancing Explained. Kellom Tomlinson. London 1735. Ref. K. 8. k. 7.
The Rudiments of Genteel Behaviour. F. Nivelon. London 1737. Ref. 1812. a. 28.
Traite sur L'Art de la Danse. N. Malpied. Paris circa 1770. Ref. 7913. f. 5.
Treatise on Dancing. F. J. Lambert. Norwich 1820. Ref. 7906. de 27.